The Neurotransmitter Solution for Migraine, Depression, and more

John A. Allocca, D.Sc., Ph.D.

Copyright © 2007, 2018
Updated 8/30/19

Published by
Allocca Biotechnology, LLC
New York
www.allocca.com

ISBN-13: 978-1984332004

ISBN-10: 1984332007

Library of Congress Control Number: 2018901961

The Neurotransmitter Solution

Table of Contents

Foreword

This book is primarily intended for healthcare practitioners. There is a significant amount of biochemistry within the book in order to show the science behind the protocol.

For the general public, ignore the biochemistry diagrams and read the text.

Introduction

Cho Seung Hui woke up one morning and was driven out of control to go on a homicidal rampage killing 32 students and faculty members. Cho Seung Hui was taking antidepressant drugs. Antidepressants have been used by the perpetrators of similar acts of violence, including the shootings at Columbine High School. There is a definite relationship between antidepressants and violent acts. Research on the drug Paxil from the Cardiff University in Britain and the Cochrane Centre in 2006 found that more than twice as many people taking it experienced a serious "hostility event" as did those taking a placebo. In the United States, labels for all antidepressants note that anxiety, agitation, panic attacks, irritability, hostility, aggressiveness, impulsivity, and mania are all possible side effects. Furthermore, what was Cho Seung Hui's diet like? Was he eating cheese?

Alone in her bed, her body twisted and distorted, Jamie cries out, "Why do I have to suffer like this?" There is no one to help her. There is no one to comfort her. She lies in her bed alone and suffering hour after hour. Although Jamie is a very pretty young woman, she can't maintain a relationship because as soon as she gets a migraine headache, her suitors run for the hills. She's gone to many doctors and specialists and she's tried many medications to no avail. She continues to suffer and suffer and suffer. Jamie is typical of millions of people who suffer from various low serotonin related disorders like migraine headaches, depression, insomnia, bipolar disorder and many more.

One day, a friend tells Jamie about a practitioner who can help her. She makes an appointment with hope and doubt at the same time. As she waits in the waiting room, she sits in silent prayer hoping for help. After what seemed like hours, she is called into the office. She immediately asks the practitioner, "Can you help me? I'm suffering from migraine headaches." The practitioner replies, "Yes, I can. But, you need to do the work. You will need to follow a comprehensive nutritional program, which begins with detoxification and bowel cleansing. Next, you need to avoid foods that cause you to lose serotonin. Then, you will need to take supplementation that will raise your of serotonin and possibly norepinephrine levels.

So, Jamie followed the program to the letter. She wouldn't even look at a piece of cheese or any other food that was on the avoid food list. And, the supplements were easy for her to take. One day about a week later, Jamie realized she didn't have a migraine headache. And, she didn't have one yesterday. And, she will probably not have one tomorrow. "Wow! I've been given my life back," said Jamie.

What is the treatment of choice? The conventional treatment uses drugs that force serotonin to remain in the neural junction. This type of treatment puts the patient at a higher risk of violent behavior. The alternative treatment is to provide the brain with the nutrients that it needs to make serotonin and norepinephrine, while following a tyramine free and possibly low tyrosine diet.

Serotonin and Norepinephrine

Serotonin

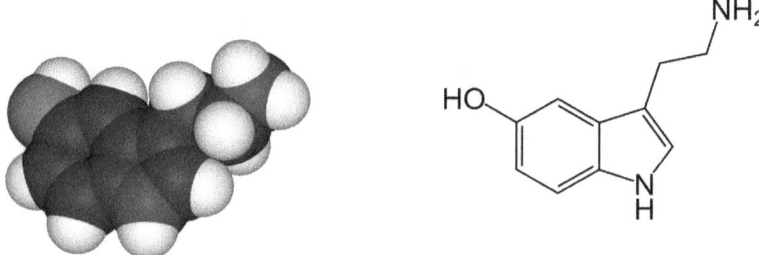

Serotonin (5-hydroxytryptamine, or 5-HT) is a monoamine neurotransmitter produced in neurons and in the gastrointestinal tract. The chemical formula for serotonin is $C_{10}H_{12}N_2O$. Serotonin cannot cross the blood-brain barrier and therefore, must be produced within the brain. About 90 percent of serotonin is produced in the gastrointestinal tract. Serotonin is stored mostly in the platelets in the blood stream. The neurons of the Raphe nuclei are the main source of serotonin release in the brain[1].

Low serotonin levels in the brain are associated with migraine headaches, depression, insomnia, bipolar syndrome, increased anger and outbursts, increased aggression, bipolar disorder, anxiety disorder, increased body temperature, moody and socially withdrawn, decreased sexuality, increased appetite for carbohydrates, irritable bowel syndrome, tinnitus, fibromyalgia, increased escape fantasies and need for change, premenstrual syndrome (PMS), and seasonal affective disorder (SAD).

Some drugs inhibit the re-uptake of serotonin making it stay in the synapse longer, which can lead to the down regulation of serotonin receptors.

> "Long-term, but not short-term, antidepressant treatment decreases the numbers of both serotonin and beta-adrenergic receptors. The decrease in the number of receptor sites is most marked for [3H] spiroperidol-labeled serotonin receptors and is characteristic for antidepressants of several classes[2]."

Serotonin is manufactured from the amino acid tryptophan. Tryptophan is the least abundant essential amino acid. An essential amino acid cannot be produced by the body and must be included in the diet. It requires an albumin carrier to

17

cross the blood-brain barrier[3] as shown in Figure 1 – Serotonin Pathways. 5-Hydroxytryptophan is the second step in serotonin production that does not require an albumin carrier to transport into the brain. 5-Hydroxytryptophan is more effective in producing serotonin than is tryptophan because it is a metabolite of tryptophan as seen in Figure 1. Common food sources of tryptophan are bananas, dried dates, milk, yogurt, cottage cheese, red meat, eggs, fish, poultry, sesame, chickpeas, sunflower seeds, pumpkin seeds, and peanuts[4].

In a research study by Johansson, et al13 a correlation between an increase in violence and reduced serotonin associated with alcoholism was seen. In the study by Linnoila, et al[14] they found low serotonin metabolite (5HIAA) levels in the cerebrospinal fluid of violent offenders, which indicates a low serotonin level in the brain. Those who attempted suicide had the lowest concentration of serotonin.

"Research on alcoholism have identified a subgroup in which the drinking problem is associated with high rates of violence, an impulsive disposition and signs of reduced serotonin functioning in the brain. The levels of serotonin and norepinephrine in the cortex were reduced[13]."

"Relationships of impulsive and nonimpulsive violent behavior to cerebrospinal fluid (CSF) monoamines and their metabolic concentrations were studied in thirty-six violent offenders. A relatively low 5-hydroxyindoleacetic acid (5HIAA) concentration was found in the CSF of impulsive violent offenders. This was not true for the offenders who had premeditated their acts. Other CSF monoamine or metabolite concentrations were not significantly different between the two groups. Of the groups studied, impulsive violent offenders who had attempted suicide had the lowest 5HIAA levels. A low CSF 5HIAA concentration may be a marker of impulsivity rather than violence[14]."

The action of serotonin, can be seen in Figure 3 – Neurotransmitter Junction.

Figure 1 – Serotonin Pathways

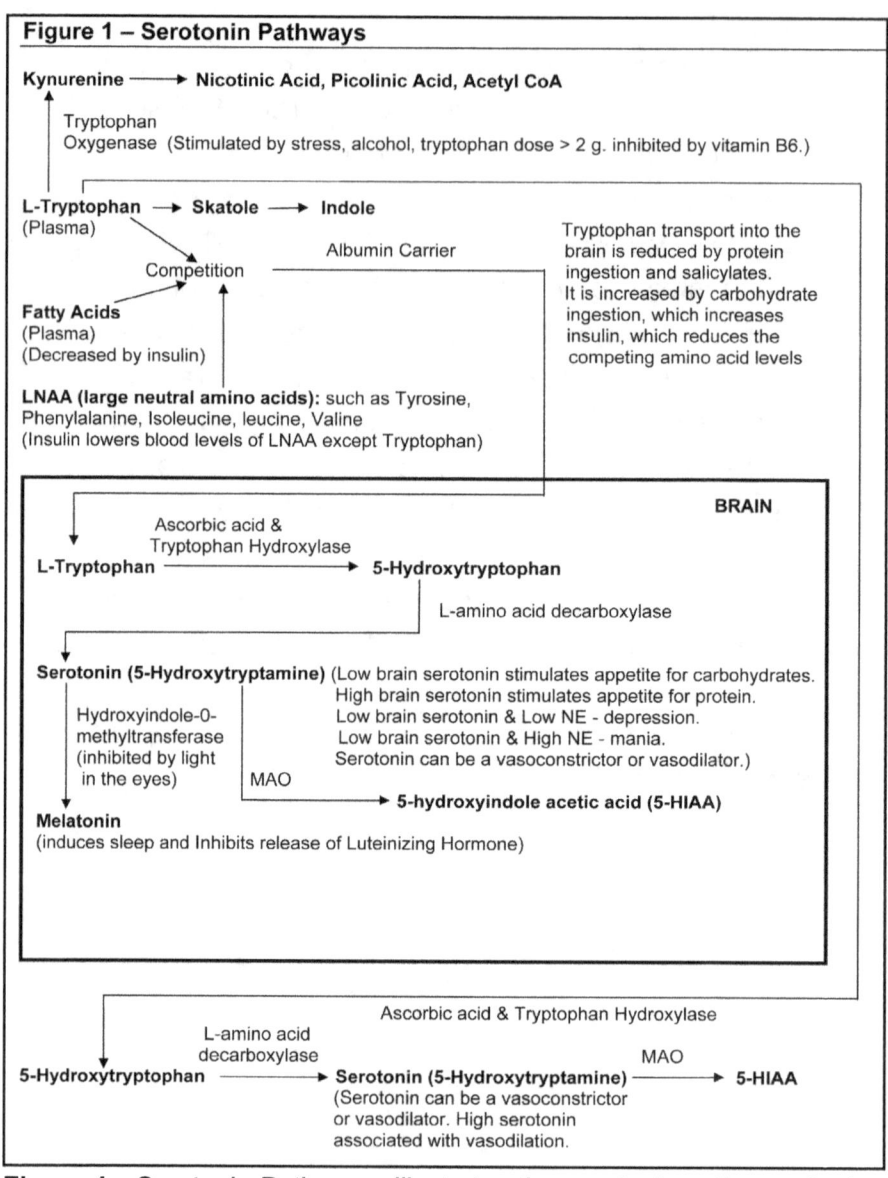

Kynurenine ──────▶ Nicotinic Acid, Picolinic Acid, Acetyl CoA

Tryptophan
Oxygenase (Stimulated by stress, alcohol, tryptophan dose > 2 g. inhibited by vitamin B6.)

L-Tryptophan ──▶ Skatole ──▶ Indole
(Plasma)

Albumin Carrier

Competition

Fatty Acids
(Plasma)
(Decreased by insulin)

Tryptophan transport into the brain is reduced by protein ingestion and salicylates. It is increased by carbohydrate ingestion, which increases insulin, which reduces the competing amino acid levels

LNAA (large neutral amino acids): such as Tyrosine, Phenylalanine, Isoleucine, leucine, Valine
(Insulin lowers blood levels of LNAA except Tryptophan)

BRAIN

Ascorbic acid &
Tryptophan Hydroxylase

L-Tryptophan ─────────────────▶ 5-Hydroxytryptophan

L-amino acid decarboxylase

Serotonin (5-Hydroxytryptamine) (Low brain serotonin stimulates appetite for carbohydrates. High brain serotonin stimulates appetite for protein. Low brain serotonin & Low NE - depression. Low brain serotonin & High NE - mania. Serotonin can be a vasoconstrictor or vasodilator.)

Hydroxyindole-0-methyltransferase (inhibited by light in the eyes)

MAO

──────▶ 5-hydroxyindole acetic acid (5-HIAA)

Melatonin
(induces sleep and Inhibits release of Luteinizing Hormone)

Ascorbic acid & Tryptophan Hydroxylase

L-amino acid
decarboxylase

MAO

5-Hydroxytryptophan ─────────▶ Serotonin (5-Hydroxytryptamine) ─────▶ 5-HIAA
(Serotonin can be a vasoconstrictor or vasodilator. High serotonin associated with vasodilation.

Figure 1 - Serotonin Pathways, illustrates the serotonin pathways in the brain and in the systemic circulation. Various enzymes control the paths to the brain or metabolism in the circulation. Tryptophan enters the brain via an albumin carrier. Proteins and fats compete for this albumin carrier. Once in the brain, tryptophan is converted to 5-Hydroxytryptophan, then into Serotonin, and Melatonin. 5-Hydroxytryptophan enters the brain via direct diffusion without an albumin carrier. If the enzyme tryptophan oxygenase is activated by stress and alcohol, tryptophan is converted into kynurenine and niacin. Tryptophan depletion in the body will result in less tryptophan to be available to enter the brain.

Norepinephrine

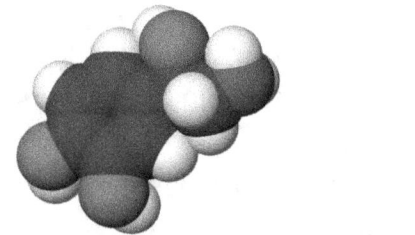

The chemical formula for norepinephrine is $C_8H_{11}NO_3$. Norepinephrine is a catecholamine that is released from the medulla of the adrenal glands as a hormone into the blood and as a neurotransmitter into the central nervous system .It is released from noradrenergic neurons during synaptic transmission. Norepinephrine is related to attention and responding actions. Along with epinephrine, norepinephrine plays an important role in the fight-or-flight response, increasing heart rate, triggering the release of glucose from energy stores, increasing wakefulness, and increasing skeletal muscle readiness[1].

Norepinephrine is released during a stressful event by activation of the locus ceruleus in the brain stem. Neurons that are activated by norepinephrine extend from the locus ceruleus to the cerebral cortex, limbic system, and the spinal cord[1].

Low norepinephrine is associated with attention-deficit/hyperactivity disorder and depression.[1,5]

Norepinephrine is manufactured from the amino acid tyrosine as shown in Figure 2 – Catecholamine Pathways.

The action of norepinephrine, as a neurotransmitter, can be seen in Figure 3 – Neurotransmitter Junction.

Tyrosine is the precursor to norepinephrine (noradrenaline), epinephrine (adrenaline), and thyroid hormones. Tyrosine can be synthesized in the body from phenylalanine, except in premature infants and in Phenylketonuria. Common food sources for phenylalanine include: pork liver, soybeans, soy products, dry skim milk, dairy, fish, meat, poultry, almonds, peanuts, brazil nuts, pecans, pumpkin seeds, sesame seeds, lima beans, chickpeas, and lentils[4]. Common food sources of tyrosine include: Meat, dairy, eggs, almonds, avocados, bananas, fish, wheat, oats, lima beans, pumpkin seeds, and sesame seeds[4].

In the study by Van Winkle, et al[16] they found that endogenous toxic metabolites interfered with neurotransmission, causing periodic depression, and overexcited synapses with excess norepinephrine causing mild anxiety to violent behavior. After the norepinephrine has been depleted, depression returned. There is a definite connection between emotions and neurotransmission. The dynamics of neurotransmitter levels in the brain need to be analyzed with respect to time. During periods of excess levels of norepinephrine in the brain, there are elevations in mood. After the norepinephrine reserves have been depleted, depression follows.

> "The continual suppression of emotions during fight or flight reactions results in atrophy and endogenous toxicosis in noradrenergic neurons. Toxic metabolites interfere with neurotransmission, causing depression. During periodic detoxification crises, excess norepinephrine floods synapses, overexcite postsynaptic neurons, and cause symptoms ranging from mild anxiety to violent behavior. When toxic metabolites, which may include excess dopamine, epinephrine, serotonin, gamma-aminobutyric acid, peptides, amino acids, and various metabolic waste products, are bound to noradrenergic receptor sites, these sites become unavailable to norepinephrine. Excitation of postsynaptic neurons is diminished and depression returns[16]."

The study by Johansson et al13 demonstrated that low levels of serotonin and norepinephrine are associated with increased violence and alcoholism. Norepinephrine is reduced by metabolizing it to epinephrine. The demand for epinephrine is stimulated during the fight or flight response, which is present during anxiety, by activating the enzyme norepinephrine methylase.

> "Research on alcoholism has identified a subgroup in which the drinking problem is associated with high rates of violence, an impulsive disposition and signs of reduced serotonin functioning in the brain. The levels of serotonin and norepinephrine in the cortex were reduced[13]."

The dynamics of neurotransmitter levels must be analyzed with respect to time. Changes in neurotransmitter levels begin with an initial reaction followed by a loss of neurotransmitter reserves if they cannot be replaced at least at the same rate by which they are depleted.

Balancing the level of norepinephrine is tricky because an increase in norepinephrine levels can lead to an increase in epinephrine levels if norepinephrine methylase is being constantly activated by a demand for epinephrine during anxiety and the fight or flight response. Norepinephrine has a stimulating effect on the stimulatory adrenergic receptors.

Epinephrine is 5-10 times more stimulating to the adrenergic receptors than norepinephrine[1]. A low level can cause depression[1] and migraine headaches[15]. A higher than normal level can cause insomnia, anxiety, etc. A very high level can cause increased aggression and perhaps violence. This statement appears to be in conflict with the study[13], in which norepinephrine levels were found to be low. This can be explained as follows. The fight or flight response calls for an increase in epinephrine. Epinephrine is metabolized from norepinephrine (see Figure 2) so that norepinephrine needs to be produced first in order to produce epinephrine. Therefore, the demand for epinephrine will initially increase the levels of norepinephrine, followed by a decrease in norepinephrine when it is metabolized to epinephrine.

If an individual is suffering from anxiety or leading a stressful or highly active lifestyle, higher than normal amounts of norepinephrine and epinephrine will be produced as a result of the fight or flight response. If that individual is following a low tyramine diet, there will be little loss of serotonin and norepinephrine. This author has found that the administration of as little as 50 mg of tyrosine to such individuals can cause insomnia and nervousness. Another factor in dosing is how much tyrosine and phenylalanine is an individual getting from food sources (see Table 1). Clinical observation and titration of tyrosine will be required to determine the proper dose of tyrosine for individuals suffering from depression and attention deficit disorder. Additional tyrosine will probably not be required for individuals suffering from anxiety, stressful lifestyles, and bipolar syndrome. Comparing the production of serotonin to norepinephrine, producing serotonin is more complicated and is more difficult than is the production of norepinephrine. Therefore, the emphasis is placed on serotonin production. Furthermore, the production of norepinephrine may not be desirable is cases of anxiety, stressful lifestyles, and bipolar syndrome.

In cases of migraine, individuals can experience a high level of stress, which converts norepinephrine to epinephrine in the fight or flight response, depleting the norepinephrine levels, particularly in the hypothalamus. If the serotonin levels are also depleted in the hypothalamus there will be a loss of vasomotor control[15]. In this case, increasing the norepinephrine levels through administration of tyrosine, could cause further conversion of norepinephrine to epinephrine in the fight or flight mode exacerbating the original problem. Therefore, titration of tyrosine on an individual basis is critical.

Chemical stimulants such as caffeine, ephedrine, pseudoephedrine, etc., can produce the fight or flight response, which can result in mania, exaggerated aggression, and perhaps violence if serotonin in the brain is low.

Mania and aggression occurs when the serotonin levels in the brain are low and the norepinephrine levels in the brain are high[15]. It appears that one of the best solutions to excessive norepinephrine and epinephrine production may be to decrease the anxiety and fight or flight response through psychotherapy, meditation, yoga, and other stress reducing modalities. If these methods are not effective or not used, maintaining an adequately high level of serotonin through diet and supplementation is vitally important.

For individuals who are chronically depressed and in attention-deficit/hyperactivity disorder, the administration of tyrosine or phenylalanine may be required. This should be done carefully and with attention to the neurotransmitter dynamics within time, to avoid promoting an increase of epinephrine.

Tyramine causes norepinephrine to be released from sympathetic nerve ending and epinephrine from the adrenal glands. Initially, this release results in increased sympathetic stimulation, which causes higher blood pressure, insomnia, increased aggression in some cases, increased glucose release, increased metabolism, inhibition of the G.I. tract, and increased cardiovascular activity. Increased sympathetic stimulation can also result in a depletion of serotonin. The final result is a depletion of norepinephrine, epinephrine, and serotonin reserves. An individual's activity, as a result of tyramine intake, may initially go from mania to depression and migraine headaches later on.

Cheese contains high amounts of tyrosine and tyramine. The high amount of tyrosine allows the norepinephrine and epinephrine levels to elevate in those who are suffering from anxiety and leading stressful and active lifestyles. The high amount of tyramine, which will be discussed in greater detail later, causes the serotonin levels to decrease. The result is mania, exaggerated aggression, and often violence. Cheddar cheese contains 42.5 mg of tyramine per ounce of cheese. An amount of 10-25 mg of tyramine can cause a severe reaction. Regardless of media advertising, cheese is not natural. It does not exist in nature. It is man-made.

If tyrosine is sufficiently increased and an individual has an adequate amount of serotonin, hyperactivity will be experienced instead of mania, exaggerated aggression, and often violence. However, this is a dangerous path as the serotonin level can drop suddenly, resulting in mania, exaggerated aggression, and often violence.

Individuals who live an anxious and stressful lifestyle, will need to follow a tyramine free and low tyrosine diet because the diet is critical to aggression and violence. Milk is relatively low in tyrosine and it contains some tryptophan. Milk also contains high biological value protein. These products may be a good source of protein for individuals who live a high stress lifestyle. In India, milk has been the primary protein source for vegetarians. Lactase should be administered along with milk to those who are lactose intolerant. If an individual is sensitive to tyrosine, milk should be taken in divided portions throughout the day.

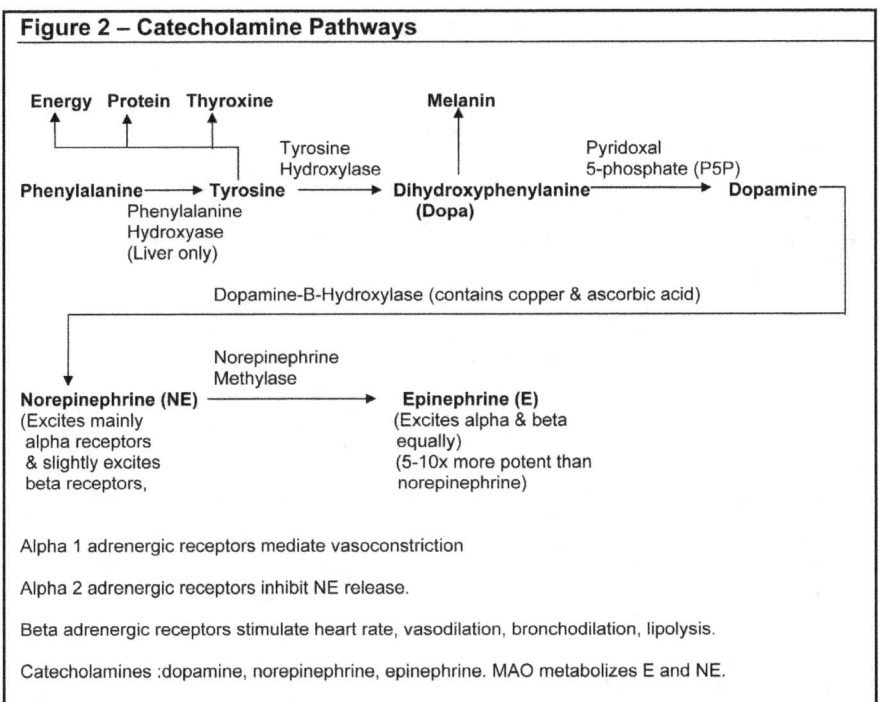

Figure 2 – Catecholamine Pathways

Energy   Protein   Thyroxine   Melanin

Tyrosine   Pyridoxal
Hydroxylase   5-phosphate (P5P)

Phenylalanine ⟶ **Tyrosine** ⟶ **Dihydroxyphenylanine** ⟶ **Dopamine**
Phenylalanine   **(Dopa)**
Hydroxyase
(Liver only)

Dopamine-B-Hydroxylase (contains copper & ascorbic acid)

Norepinephrine
Methylase

Norepinephrine (NE) ⟶ **Epinephrine (E)**
(Excites mainly   (Excites alpha & beta
alpha receptors   equally)
& slightly excites   (5-10x more potent than
beta receptors,   norepinephrine)

Alpha 1 adrenergic receptors mediate vasoconstriction

Alpha 2 adrenergic receptors inhibit NE release.

Beta adrenergic receptors stimulate heart rate, vasodilation, bronchodilation, lipolysis.

Catecholamines :dopamine, norepinephrine, epinephrine. MAO metabolizes E and NE.

Figure 2 - Catecholamine Pathways, illustrates the dopamine, norepinephrine, and epinephrine pathways. Norepinephrine is found low in depression and in migraine.

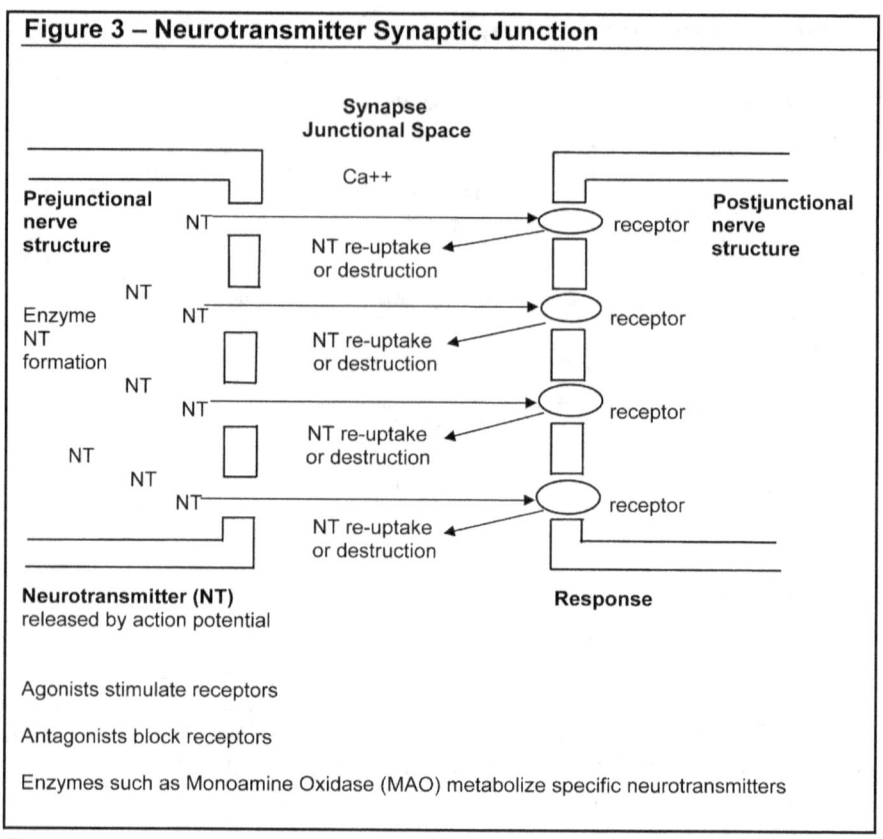

Figure 3 – Neurotransmitter Synaptic Junction

Synapse
Junctional Space

Ca++

Prejunctional nerve structure

NT ─────────► receptor   Postjunctional nerve structure

NT re-uptake or destruction

NT

Enzyme NT formation

NT ─────────► receptor

NT re-uptake or destruction

NT

NT ─────────► receptor

NT re-uptake or destruction

NT

NT

NT ─────────► receptor

NT re-uptake or destruction

Neurotransmitter (NT)
released by action potential

Response

Agonists stimulate receptors

Antagonists block receptors

Enzymes such as Monoamine Oxidase (MAO) metabolize specific neurotransmitters

Figure 3 - Neurotransmitter Synaptic Junction, illustrates the paths of neurotransmitters in the prejunctional nerve across the synaptic junction to the receptors in the postjunctional nerve. Agonists are substances that stimulate receptors and Antagonists block them. After transmission, neurotransmitters are either taken up by the prejunctional nerve and recycled or metabolized, or they are metabolized in or near the junctional space.

Serotonin and Norepinephrine Related Disorders

Migraine Headaches, Depression, and Insomnia

Migraine is characterized by a loss of vasomotor control, which is due to a loss of or low level of serotonin and norepinephrine particularly in the hypothalamus. This results in vascular dilation, which causes the associated throbbing pain. This loss of neurotransmitters can occur as a result of several factors, such as chemicals that cause the loss of neurotransmitters, allergic reactions, inflammation, poor absorption of precursors into the brain, lack of precursors, or poor metabolism of precursors in the brain.

The Migraine Syndrome may begin in childhood, adolescence or early adult life and continue to reoccur at periodic intervals. There are two major classifications of migraine headaches, with and without visual disturbances. The migraine with visual disturbances, which is usually the most severe, is characterized by a visual disturbance, numbness on one side of the body or limb, and/or slight speech abnormality. These symptoms, referred to as the "aura," will diminish as a headache, nausea, vomiting etc. become more pronounced.

The visual disturbance may last anywhere from 5 minutes to 30 minutes. As the visual disturbance slowly disappears, it gives way to boring pain generalized or localized in one area of the head. The pain will increase in intensity and acquire a throbbing character. The throbbing characteristic may be intensified by stooping and by all forms of exertion, light, or sound. If you lie down the intensity may be increased, and it is slightly reduced when sitting upright. This is due to an increase of pressure in the head when lying down and a decrease when sitting up. In many cases, the pain may extend down to the neck.

The throbbing pain and visual disturbances are often accompanied by abdominal pains and vomiting. Almost all migraine sufferers experience nausea to some extent. As vomiting occurs, so does sweating and chills due to the severe fluid and nutrient depletion. Diarrhea, often preceded by constipation, will usually occur about the same time as the nausea and/or vomiting.

During a migraine attack, one will undergo a state of mental confusion, altered consciousness, and may experience a state of euphoria. Along with this confusion and euphoria is the constant throbbing of pain, which will not stop. During the headache, one may experience mood changes with feelings of being rejected and often seriously depressed. At times one may be unsociable, rejecting companionship or the presence of others, becoming irritable and rejecting any demand to make a decision. Migraine attacks will vary in duration and intensity. A Migraine attack can last from hours to days. After an attack one may feel relaxed, in good spirits, be filled with energy and drive, enthusiastic about work, and sometimes overly active. There may be a feeling of physical depletion for a day or two, especially if there has been a great deal of vomiting or diarrhea. The frequency of migraine attacks vary from daily to only a few times in a lifetime. Between attacks there are almost no symptoms with the exception of the "type A" personality, irritability, and depression.

Imbalances in brain chemistry, particularly neurotransmitter levels, have a large range of effects on emotions, behavior, and brain circulation. Neurotransmitters are chemical substances that pass signals between nerves.

Serotonin and norepinephrine are the two main neurotransmitters used in the brain to control the size of blood vessels as well as other functions. These neurotransmitter levels can be diminished by allergic reactions, inflammation, poor absorption of nutrients into the brain, poor metabolism of nutrients in the brain, chemicals that deplete them, excessive depletion (over usage) lowering them or because there are not enough nutrients in the brain to produce more. Congestive bowel toxicity and intestinal dysbiosis play a major role in producing toxins. Migraine, depression, and insomnia have similar mechanisms and pathways, all resulting from a loss of serotonin and norepinephrine[15].

Migraine, depression, and insomnia have similar mechanisms and pathways, all resulting from a loss of serotonin and norepinephrine[15].

The loss of serotonin and norepinephrine may be quantified in three stages[15]. Stage 1 is the first level below normal. Insomnia will be experienced during Stage 1 because there is not enough serotonin to produce melatonin, which is required for sleep. Insomnia may also occur as a result of excessive epinephrine, which is caused by converting norepinephrine to epinephrine as a result of anxiety. Stage 2 is the next level below Stage 1. When the serotonin and norepinephrine levels fall to Stage 2, depression will be experienced. Stage 3 is the next level below Stage 2. When the serotonin and norepinephrine levels fall to Stage 3, there is a loss of vasomotor control and the migraine headache results.

The diameter of the blood vessels in the head as well as other functions, are controlled by signals transmitted along nerves. Neurotransmitters are chemical substances that pass signals along nerves. Normally, a part of the brain sends signals along the nerves to keep the blood vessels in the head at a constant size. However, if there are not enough neurotransmitters in the brain to control the size of the blood vessels in the head, they will continually enlarge until they cannot stretch any longer. The enlarged blood vessels will create a tremendous amount of pain, hence the migraine headache. It has been thought that there are two mechanisms of vasomotor control, vasodilation and vasoconstriction. However, this author believes there is only one mechanism, vasoconstriction. Blood vessels dilate from a lack of vasoconstriction and the pressure inside the vessel. Excessive vasoconstriction can also deplete serotonin and norepinephrine.

A study by Eklundh, T et al, Aviat Space Environ Med. 2000 Nov;71(11):1131-6, shows that atmospheric pressure influences increased CSF levels of monoamine oxidase and cholecystokinin peptides. Monoamine oxidase metabolizes serotonin, which explains why people experience depression and migraine headaches during periods of low barometric pressure associated with weather storms.

Symptoms of migraine include:

- Throbbing or intense pain on one side or front and rear of head or eye
- Headache preceded by a short period of depression, irritability, or restlessness
- Headache preceded by visual flashing zig-zag lines
- Headache preceded by other visual disturbances
- Visual disturbances disappear shortly after headache begins
- Nausea associated with headache
- Sensitive to light, especially during headache
- Sensitive to noise, especially during headache
- Extremities are cold before and during headache
- Family history of migraine
- Difficulty with speech before headache
- Intensity of headache increases when lying down
- Often prefer seclusion

Migraine is often misdiagnosed as a severe headache. The hemicranial (one side of the head) throbbing pain differentiates migraine from tension headaches.

Chronic Migraine Diagnostic Criteria

Chronic migraine: headache (not attributable to another disorder) on => 15 days/month for > 3 months fulfilling the following criteria for migraine:

At least 2 of the following:
> 1. unilateral location
> 2. pulsating quality
> 3. moderate/severe pain intensity
> 4. aggravation by routine physical activity

At least 1 of the following:
> 1. nausea and/or vomiting
> 2. photophobia and phonophobia

International Classification of Headache Disorders, 2nd ed. ICHD-II 1.5.1 & 1.6.5

Note: many people and healthcare practitioners do not understand the diagnostic criteria for migraine. They often believe that a migraine headache is a "severe headache" when it may actually be a sinus or tension headache. The word "migraine" comes from the Greek word "hemikrania", which means "pain on one side of the head."

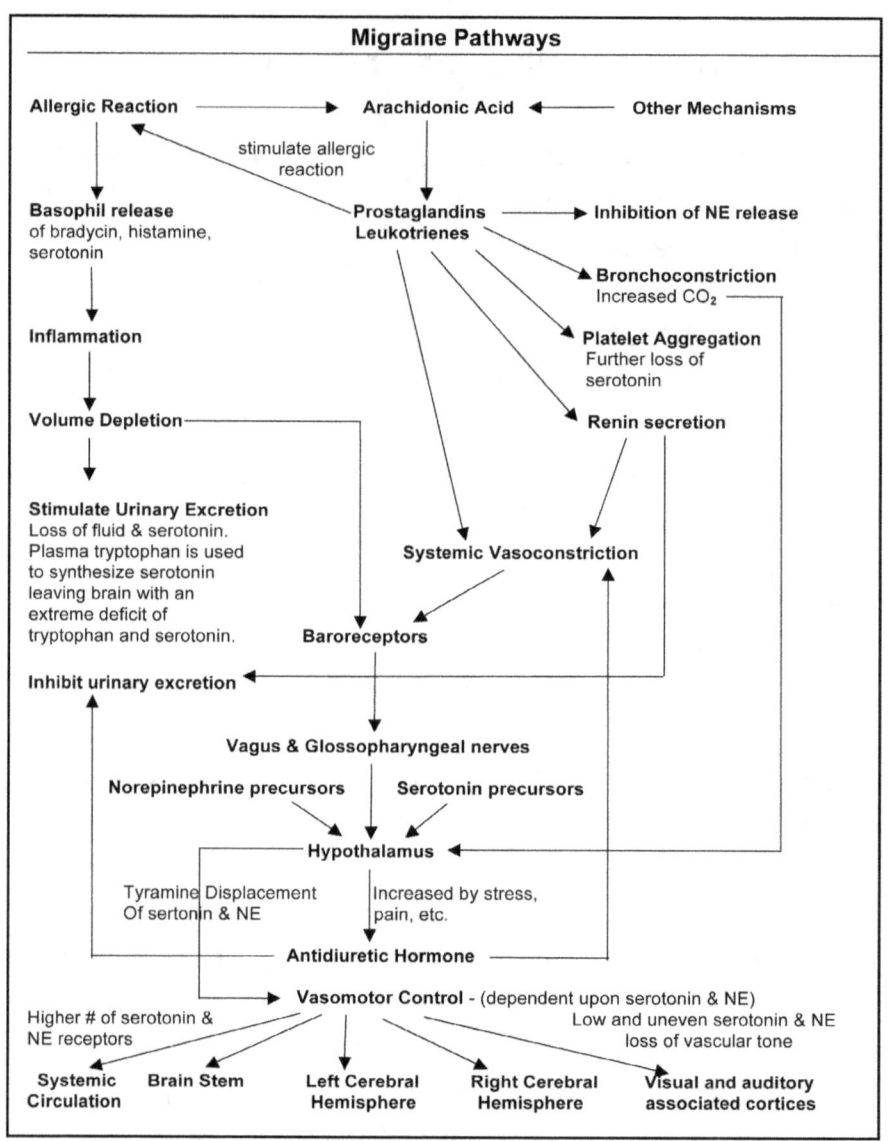

Migraine Pathways

Figure 4 - Migraine Pathways, illustrates the many pathways that trigger a migraine attack. Most of the pathways lead to inflammation and loss of serotonin and norepinephrine. The loss of serotonin and norepinephrine in the brain results in a loss of vasomotor control by the hypothalamus of various circulatory paths in the brain. The resulting loss of vasomotor control causes the arteries to dilate (loses its ability to constrict). This dilation may occur to some degree systemically.

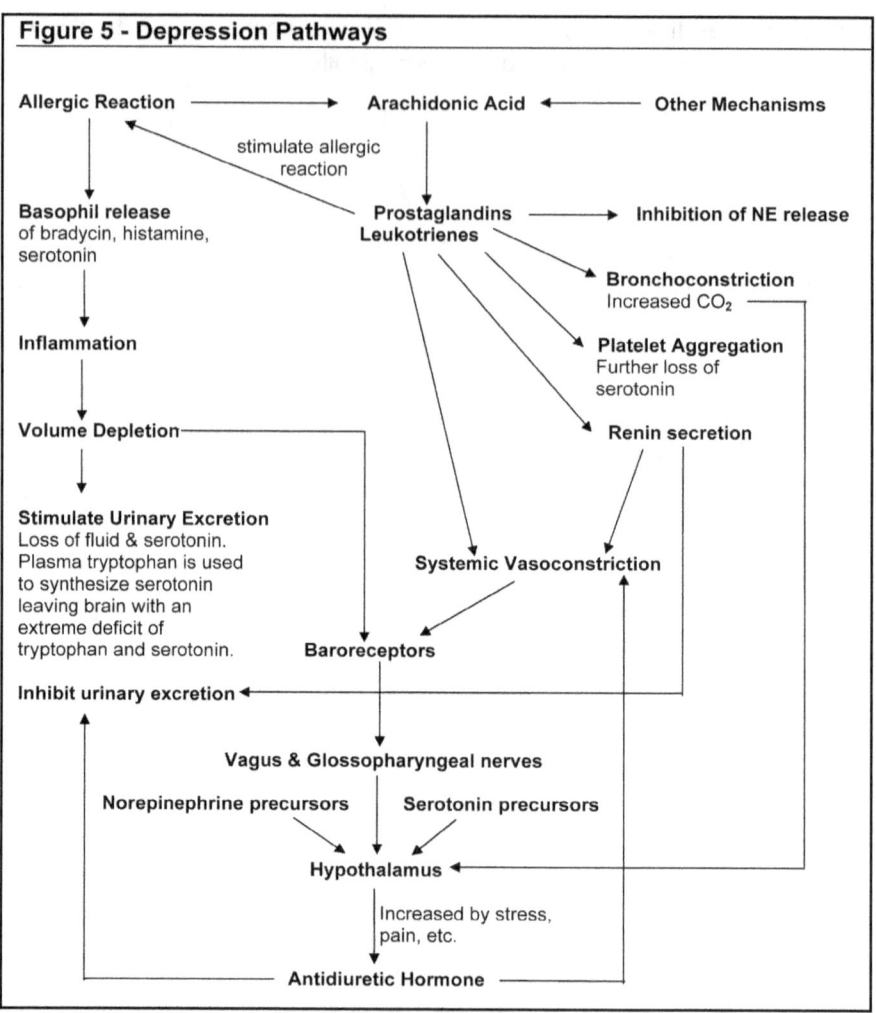

Figure 5 - Depression Pathways

Figure 5 - Depression Pathways, is similar to the Migraine Pathways diagram without the vasomotor control mechanisms. This diagram illustrates the many pathways that can be initiated to cause depression. Most of the pathways lead to inflammation and loss of serotonin.

Anger, Violence, and Bipolar Syndrome

Many aspects of this section were already covered in the "Serotonin and Norepinephrine" section.

The symptoms of bipolar syndrome are not so easily noticed. Bipolar syndrome is often characterized by an individual who is quiet or depressed one moment, then exhibits mania or rage the next moment.

"Many people, especially children have poor diets resulting from high toxin levels and low nutrient levels, which can lead to low serotonin levels in the brain. Low levels of serotonin and low levels of norepinephrine can cause depression. Consequently, they will experience depression and fatigue and pursue stimulants such as coffee and soft drinks containing high amounts of caffeine. The caffeine causes an increase in epinephrine, and norepinephrine levels in the brain. When there is low serotonin and high norepinephrine levels in the brain, an individual may exhibit manic behavior and when high enough, violence"[15]. Furthermore, if that individual eats cheese, their serotonin level will drop and their norepinephrine level will rise, leading to increased aggression and violence.

As previously discussed, the dynamics of neurotransmitter levels must be analyzed with respect to time. Changes in neurotransmitter levels begin with an initial reaction followed by a loss of neurotransmitter reserves if they cannot be replaced at the same rate by which they are depleted.

In the study by Barbara Stanley, et al[17], their findings of reduced serotonin metabolite (5-HIAA) levels and aggression supports and extends previous studies linking low cerebrospinal fluid 5-HIAA levels to aggression in impulsive murderers, arsonists, and individuals convicted of infanticide, as well as research showing that recidivists have lower levels of the serotonin metabolite than non-recidivists.

"A new study[17] adds to evidence linking reduced serotonin levels to aggression even in the absence of suicidal tendencies. Barbara Stanley et al, measured cerebrospinal fluid levels of the serotonin metabolite 5-hydroxyindoleacetic acid (5-HIAA) in 64 psychiatric patients with a range of disorders including bipolar disorder, major depressive or dysthymic disorder, schizophrenia, and schizoaffective disorder. None had a history of suicidal behavior. The subjects were divided into two groups, based on high or low scores on measures of adult aggression. When mean CSF 5-HIAA levels of the two groups were compared, Stanley et al. say, the aggressive group was found to have significantly lower CSF 5-HIAA concentrations than the non-aggressive group"[18]

The study by Davidson, Richard J, et al[19], as well as other studies, shows that the prefrontal cortex area of the brain is responsible for the control of aggression and violent behavior. It appears that this area of the brain, when working properly, inhibits aggression and violence. Therefore, a low level of serotonin in this area of the brain will reduce an individual's ability to inhibit aggressive and violent behavior.

> "Emotion is normally regulated in the human brain by a complex circuit consisting of the orbital frontal cortex, amygdala, anterior cingulate cortex, and several other interconnected regions. There are both genetic and environmental contributions to the structure and function of this circuitry. We posit that impulsive aggression and violence arise as a consequence of faulty emotion regulation. Indeed, the prefrontal cortex receives a major serotonergic projection, which is dysfunctional in individuals who show impulsive violence. Individuals vulnerable to faulty regulation of negative emotion are at risk for violence and aggression. Research on the neural circuitry of emotion regulation suggests new avenues of intervention for such at-risk populations."[19]

Research[20] has demonstrated that men with a deficiency in the prefrontal cortex of their brain are prone to rage and violence. Brain imaging showed a lack of nerve cells in the prefrontal cortex of the brains in the men, who had all committed serious, violent crimes and had psychopathic personalities. The prefrontal cortex is an area of the brain that plays a key role in children's ability to learn to feel remorse, conscience and social sensitivity. Therefore, a low level of serotonin in the prefrontal cortex of the brain will reduce an individual's ability to inhibit aggressive and violent behavior.

"Many people have poor diets resulting from high toxin levels and low nutrient levels, which can lead to low serotonin levels in the brain. Low levels of serotonin and low levels of norepinephrine can cause depression. Consequently, they will experience depression and fatigue and pursue stimulants such as coffee and soft drinks containing high amounts of caffeine. The caffeine causes an increase in cortisol, epinephrine, and norepinephrine levels in the brain. When there is low serotonin and high norepinephrine levels in the brain, an individual may exhibit anxious, aggressive, manic, behavior, possibly with outbursts, and when high enough, violence. This type of behavior may be augmented if there is little serotonin in the prefrontal cortex of the brain. In milder cases, the individual may be moody and socially withdrawn. They may also experience an increase in escape fantasies and a need for change."[15]

"With the availability of new functional and structural neuroimaging techniques, researchers have begun to localize brain areas that may be dysfunctional in offenders who are aggressive and violent. Our review of 17 neuroimaging studies reveals that the areas associated with aggressive and/or violent behavioral histories, particularly impulsive acts, are located in the prefrontal cortex and the medial temporal regions. These findings are explained in the context of negative emotion regulation, and suggestions are provided concerning how such findings may affect future theoretical frameworks in criminology, crime prevention efforts, and the functioning of the criminal justice system[11]."

"Humans are endowed with a natural sense of fairness that permeates social perceptions and interactions. This moral stance is so ubiquitous that we may not notice it as a fundamental component of daily decision making and in the workings of many legal, political, and social systems. Using functional magnetic resonance imaging and a passive visual task, we show that both basic and moral emotions activate the amygdala, thalamus, and upper midbrain. The orbital and medial prefrontal cortex and the superior temporal sulcus are also recruited by viewing scenes evocative of moral emotions. Our results indicate that the orbital and medial sectors of the prefrontal cortex and the superior temporal sulcus region, which are critical regions for social behavior and perception, play a central role in moral appraisals. We suggest that the automatic tagging of ordinary social events with moral values may be an important mechanism for implicit social behaviors in humans[12]."

Decreased Sexuality

Nitric oxide, serotonin, dopamine, epinephrine, and norepinephrine, are just a few of the neurotransmitters and neuropeptides involved in sexual activity. Serotonin's causes the constriction of smooth muscles in the genitals, and peripheral nerve function, which increases the rate and force of the muscle's contractions during sexual activity.[22]. Levels of norepinephrine in the brain increase significantly with arousal and sexual activity in men as well as in women[22]. Low serotonin and low epinephrine will lead to depression and a loss of libido[15].

In the study, "Dopamine and serotonin: influences on male sexual behavior," by Hull EM, et al[21], dopamine facilitates sexual motivation while the effects of serotonin has mixed effects being either inhibition or stimulation.

> "Steroid hormones regulate sexual behavior primarily by slow, genomically mediated effects. These effects are realized, in part, by enhancing the processing of relevant sensory stimuli, altering the synthesis, release, and/or receptors for neurotransmitters in integrative areas, and increasing the responsiveness of appropriate motor outputs. Dopamine has facilitative effects on sexual motivation, copulatory proficiency, and genital reflexes.

Dopamine in the nigrostriatal tract influences motor activity; in the mesolimbic tract it activates numerous motivated behaviors, including copulation; in the medial preoptic area (MPOA) it controls genital reflexes, copulatory patterns, and specifically sexual motivation. Testosterone increases nitric oxide synthase in the MPOA; nitric oxide increases basal and female-stimulated dopamine release, which in turn facilitates copulation and genital reflexes. Serotonin (5-HT) is primarily inhibitory, although stimulation of 5-HT(2C) receptors increases erections and inhibits ejaculation, whereas stimulation of 5-HT(1A) receptors has the opposite effects: facilitation of ejaculation and, in some circumstances, inhibition of erection. 5-HT is released in the anterior lateral hypothalamus at the time of ejaculation. Microinjections of selective serotonin reuptake inhibitors there delay the onset of copulation and delay ejaculation after copulation begins. One means for this inhibition is a decrease in dopamine release in the mesolimbic tract."[21]

Increased Body Temperature

Body temperature is regulated by the hypothalamus. If the hypothalamus is low in serotonin, it can raise body temperature. A study[23] by J.L. Rausch, et al, demonstrated that there was a significantly higher body temperature in depressed patients.

Increased Appetite for Carbohydrates

As seen in Figure 1 – Serotonin Pathways, an albumin carrier is required to transport tryptophan across the blood-brain barrier. Fatty acids and large neutral amino acids will compete for the albumin carrier. A low brain serotonin level stimulates the body's appetite for carbohydrates in order to facilitate the transport of tryptophan into the brain. High brain serotonin level stimulates appetite for protein in order to inhibit the transport of tryptophan into the brain. The study by Heath TP, et al[24], shows that enhancing serotonin significantly reduces the taste for sucrose. Enhancing norepinephrine significantly reduced the taste for bitters and salt. They also found that the anxiety level was also related to taste perception.

> "Circumstances in which serotonin (5-HT) and noradrenaline (NA) are altered, such as in anxiety or depression, are associated with taste disturbances, indicating the importance of these transmitters in the determination of taste thresholds in health and disease. In this study, we show for the first time that human taste thresholds are plastic and are lowered by modulation of systemic monoamines. Measurement of taste function in healthy humans before and after a 5-HT reuptake inhibitor, NA reuptake inhibitor, or placebo

showed that enhancing 5-HT significantly reduced the sucrose taste threshold by 27% and the quinine taste threshold by 53%. In contrast, enhancing NA significantly reduced bitter taste threshold by 39% and sour threshold by 22%. In addition, the anxiety level was positively correlated with bitter and salt taste thresholds. We show that 5-HT and NA participate in setting taste thresholds, that human taste in normal healthy subjects is plastic, and that modulation of these neurotransmitters has distinct effects on different taste modalities. We present a model to explain these findings. In addition, we show that the general anxiety level is directly related to taste perception, suggesting that altered taste and appetite seen in affective disorders may reflect an actual change in the gustatory system."[24]

Irritable Bowel Syndrome

Recent research has demonstrated that low serotonin levels are related to poor gastrointestinal functioning. People with Irritable Bowel Syndrome have diminished receptor activity in the cells that line the inside of the bowel, causing low levels of serotonin to exist in the GI tract. As a result, people with Irritable Bowel Syndrome experience problems with bowel movement, motility, and sensation and having more sensitive pain receptors in their GI tract. People who suffer from Irritable Bowel Syndrome often suffer from depression and anxiety. The study by Chua AS, et al[25], shows that serotonin can decrease gastric emptying and appetite.

> "Symptoms of functional dyspepsia are characterized by upper abdominal discomfort or pain, early satiety, postprandial fullness, bloating, nausea and vomiting. It is a chronic disorder, with symptoms more than 3 mo per year, and no evidence of organic diseases. Dysfunctional motility, altered visceral sensation, and psychosocial factors have all been identified as major pathophysiological mechanisms. It is believed that these pathophysiological mechanisms interact to produce the observed symptoms. Dyspepsia has been categorized into three subgroups based on dominant symptoms. Dysmotility-like

dyspepsia describes a subgroup of patients whose symptom complex is usually related to a gastric sensorimotor dysfunction. The brain-gut peptide cholecystokinin (CCK) and serotonin (5-HT) share certain physiological effects. Both have been shown to decrease gastric emptying and affect satiety. Furthermore the CCK induced anorexia depended on serotonergic functions probably acting via central pathways. We believe that abnormalities of central serotonergic receptors functioning together with a hyper responsiveness to CCK or their interactions may be responsible for the genesis of symptoms in functional dyspepsia (FD)."[25]

According to the study by van Lelyveld N, et al[26], there is a higher serotonin functioning in the duodenum than the stomach.

"The aim of this study was to increase the understanding of the role of serotonergic signaling in normal gastroduodenal function at a molecular level. Mucosal biopsy specimens were collected from the fundus, antrum and duodenum of 11 healthy subjects. Serotonin transport protein expression was 19-fold higher in the duodenum compared with the antrum and 457-fold higher compared with the fundus ($P < 0.001$). Tryptophan hydroxylase-1 expression was lower in the duodenum compared with the antrum and fundus (regional differences -2.3 and -3.6, respectively). The 5-HT(4) receptor and the 5-HT(3C) and 5-HT(3E) receptor subunits were more abundantly expressed in duodenum compared with the stomach (P < 0.001). The larger number of 5-HT-positive cells, the higher expression of 5-HT(3) and 5-HT(4) receptors, and in particularly the higher uptake capacity of 5-HT in the duodenum, point out to a more prominent role of serotonergic signalling at the mucosal level in the duodenum compared with the stomach."[26]

The study by Shufflebotham J, et al[27], shows the correlation between low serotonin and irritable bowel syndrome.

"OBJECTIVES: To assess the effect of acute changes in serotonin (5-HT) synthesis using the acute tryptophan depletion (ATD) paradigm on gastrointestinal (GI) and mood symptoms in irritable bowel syndrome (IBS). METHODS: In a randomized double-blind crossover study, 29 subjects (18 patients with ROME II defined IBS and 11 age-matched controls) were studied under ATD and acute tryptophan increase (ATI) conditions. GI symptoms, mood and anxiety ratings, as well as plasma tryptophan concentrations were measured. RESULTS: Total (and free) plasma tryptophan concentrations decreased on the ATD day in patients (73%[82%]) and controls (73%[80%]), and increased on the ATI day in patients (59%[143%]) and controls (61%[381%]). Compared with the ATD day, IBS patients reported more GI symptoms on the ATI day at +210 ($p < 0.001$) and at +270 ($p < 0.05$) min post drink. IBS patients also reported less anxiety on the ATI day compared with the ATD day at +270 min ($p < 0.001$). ATD and ATI did not affect these ratings in control participants. IBS patients had a lower mood compared with controls ($p < 0.05$), but this did not differ between the ATI and ATD days in either group. CONCLUSIONS: IBS patients' GI and anxiety responses to changes in tryptophan load differ from controls. This suggests a difference in serotonergic functioning between these two groups and provides evidence to support the hypothesis that 5-HT dysfunction is involved in IBS[27].

Tinnitus

In reviewing the serotonin pathways, tryptophan is converted to serotonin. Serotonin is converted to melatonin by activation of the enzyme hydroxyindole-o-methyltransferase, which is inhibited by light in the eyes[15].

A clinical study[28] was conducted at the Shea Ear Clinic in Sarasota, FL. They tested 3 mg of melatonin on tinnitus patients for one month. They found that those people who did not have trouble sleeping were not greatly benefited by the melatonin, which is derived from serotonin. However, of the people who had difficulty sleeping, 47% reported an overall improvement in their tinnitus.

The study by Megwalu UC, et al[29], showed that melatonin clearly improves tinnitus, especially in individuals with poor sleep.

"GOAL: To determine if melatonin improves tinnitus and if this improvement is related to improvement in sleep. STUDY DESIGN AND SETTING: Prospective open-label study of 24 patients with tinnitus. The patients took 3 mg of melatonin per day for 4 weeks, followed by 4 weeks of observation. The Tinnitus Handicap Inventory (THI) and the Pittsburgh Sleep Quality Index (PSQI) were administered.

RESULTS: The mean THI score decreased significantly between weeks 0 and 4, and between weeks 0 and 8. The mean PSQI significantly decreased between weeks 0 and 4 ($P < 0.0001$), and between weeks 0 and 8 ($P = 0.0003$). The change in PSQI was significantly associated with the change in THI between weeks 0 and 4. The change in PSQI was not significantly associated with the change in THI between weeks 0 and 8. The change in the PSQI in the first 4 weeks was associated with the initial PSQI. There was no association between the initial THI and the change in the THI in the first 4 weeks. CONCLUSION: Melatonin use is associated with improvement of tinnitus and sleep. There was an association between the amount of improvement in sleep and tinnitus. The impact of melatonin on sleep was greatest among patients with the worst sleep quality, but its impact on tinnitus was not associated with the severity of the tinnitus. SIGNIFICANCE: Melatonin may be a safe treatment for patients with idiopathic tinnitus, especially those with sleep disturbance due to tinnitus."[29]

Fibromyalgia

Serotonin levels are normally lower in women than men, which makes women more likely to develop fibromyalgia. Statistically, women are much more likely to be diagnosed with fibromyalgia than are men. Fibromyalgia is usually worse at night. Serotonin normally reduces the intensity of pain signals.

In the study by Juhl JH, et al[30], the researchers studied the evidence from multiple sources and concluded that serotonin is low in fibromyalgia patients and that improvement was seen with supplementation with L-tryptophan or 5-hydroxytryptophan.

> "Fibromyalgia syndrome is a musculoskeletal pain and fatigue disorder manifested by diffuse myalgia, localized areas of tenderness, fatigue, lowered pain thresholds, and nonrestorative sleep. Evidence from multiple sources support the concept of decreased flux through the serotonin pathway in fibromyalgia patients. Serotonin substrate supplementation, via L-tryptophan or 5-hydroxytryptophan (5-HTP), has been shown to improve symptoms of depression, anxiety, insomnia and somatic pains in a variety of patient cohorts. Identification of low serum tryptophan and

serotonin levels may be a simple way to identify persons who will respond well to this approach."[30]

"Although disturbances in the musculoskeletal system, in the neuroendocrine system and in the central nervous system (CNS) have been implicated in the pathophysiology of fibromyalgia syndrome (FMS), the primary mechanisms underlying the etiopathogenesis of FMS remain elusive. It has been postulated that disturbances in serotonin metabolism and transmission, along with disturbances in several other chemical pain mediators, are present in patients with FMS. In this article we review published studies on the pathophysiological role of serotonin in FMS. Although studies that indirectly measured the function of serotonin in the CNS in FMS revealed some abnormalities in the metabolism and transmission of serotonin, the role of serotonin in the pathophysiology of syndrome remains inconclusive and warrants more studies."[31]

Birdsall TC, et al[32], has shown that 5-Hydroxytryptophan, unlike tryptophan, does not require an albumin carrier to transport into the brain. They also found that 5-Hydroxytryptophan cannot be shunted into niacin like tryptophan does. This is extremely significant clinically because patients can take 5-Hydroxytryptophan with food in their stomach and achieve higher levels in the brain than with tryptophan.

"5-Hydroxytryptophan (5-HTP) is the intermediate metabolite of the essential amino acid L-tryptophan (LT) in the biosynthesis of serotonin. Intestinal absorption of 5-HTP does not require the presence of a transport molecule, and is not affected by the presence of other amino acids; therefore it may be taken with meals without reducing its effectiveness. Unlike LT, 5-HTP cannot be shunted into niacin or protein production. Therapeutic use of 5-HTP bypasses the conversion of LT into 5-HTP by the enzyme tryptophan hydroxylase, which is the rate-limiting step in the synthesis of serotonin. 5-HTP is well absorbed from an oral dose, with about 70 percent ending up in the bloodstream. It easily crosses the blood-brain barrier and effectively increases central nervous system (CNS) synthesis of serotonin. In the CNS, serotonin levels have been implicated in the regulation of sleep, depression, anxiety, aggression, appetite, temperature, sexual behaviour, and pain sensation. Therapeutic administration of 5-HTP has been shown to be effective in treating a wide variety of conditions, including depression, fibromyalgia, binge eating associated with obesity, chronic headaches, and insomnia."[32]

Premenstrual Syndrome (PMS)

PMS can also affect women who have had their uterus removed. PMS relates to the enrichment of the uterine lining in preparation for arrival of a fertilized egg. This phase of the lining's growth is associated with increased levels of progesterone at the time when an ovary releases its egg. The increased progesterone may decrease levels of serotonin in the brain. This may be the reason for the agitation, mood swings, restlessness, and food cravings.

Steinberg S, et al[33], has shown the therapeutic effects of increasing serotonin in premenstrual syndrome using the Visual Analog Mood Scale. The results also indicate that increasing L-tryptophan, which in turn increases serotonin levels, elevates the mood and makes people feel better.

> "In a randomized controlled clinical trial, 37 patients with premenstrual dysphoric disorder were treated with L-tryptophan 6 g per day and 34 were given placebo. The treatments were given under double-blind conditions for 17 days, from the time of ovulation to the third day of menstruation, during three consecutive cycles. Visual Analog Mood Scales revealed a significant ($p = 0.004$) therapeutic effect of L-tryptophan relative to placebo for the cluster of mood symptoms comprising the items

dysphoria, mood swings, tension and irritability. These results suggest that increasing serotonin synthesis during the late luteal phase of the menstrual cycle is therapeutic in patients with premenstrual dysphoric disorder."[33]

Menkes DB, et al[34], suppressed serotonin by tryptophan depletion in a study of 16 women with premenstrual syndrome. They found a significant aggravation of symptoms.

> "The dietary technique of acute tryptophan depletion was used to suppress brain serotonin synthesis in 16 women with documented premenstrual syndrome. Each subject was tested at distinct phases of each of two menstrual cycles. Baseline amino acid levels did not vary across the menstrual cycle, except for tyrosine which showed a significant premenstrual decrement. Compared to a sham procedure, actual tryptophan depletion caused a significant aggravation of premenstrual symptoms, particularly irritability. Symptom magnitude was correlated with diminution of tryptophan relative to other amino acids. This result supports other evidence implicating serotonin in premenstrual syndrome."[34]

Seasonal Affective Disorder (SAD)

Medical research has shown that seasonal affective disorder is caused by the decreased exposure to sunlight during the fall and winter months. Light inhibits the activity of hydroxytryptamine-o-methyltransferase, which converts serotonin to melatonin[15]. Without adequate sunlight, serotonin may be lost by being converted to melatonin. Melatonin is a hormone that aids the body in sleeping.

Miller AL, et al[35], used light therapy in their study to decrease the levels of melatonin in northern latitudes. As mentioned earlier, light inhibits the activity of hydroxytryptamine-o-methyltransferase, which converts serotonin to melatonin[15].

> "There is much more seasonal difference in higher latitudes than in lower latitudes. In a significant portion of the population of the northern United States, the shorter days of fall and winter precipitate a syndrome that can consist of depression, fatigue, hypersomnolence, hyperphagia, carbohydrate craving, weight gain, and loss of libido. If these symptoms persist in the winter, abate as the days grow longer, and disappear in the summer, the diagnosis of seasonal affective disorder (SAD) can be made. Many hypotheses exist regarding the biochemical

mechanisms behind the predisposition toward this disease, including circadian phase shifting, abnormal pineal melatonin secretion, and abnormal serotonin synthesis. Although the mechanism(s) behind this disease is not fully known, one treatment appears to address each of the theories. Light therapy is a natural, non-invasive, effective, well-researched method of treatment for SAD. Various light temperatures and times of administration of light therapy have been studied, and a combination of morning and evening exposure appears to offer the best efficacy. Other natural methods of treatment have been studied, including L-tryptophan, Hypericum perforatum (St. John's wort), and melatonin."[35]

Neumeister A, et al[36], found that not all patients with seasonal affective disorder experience depression every winter. However, they did find a correlation between tryptophan and depression in patients with seasonal affective disorder, even in the summer. This study suggests that the serotonin level is low in seasonal affective disorder during times of depression. Therefore, increasing the serotonin level by tryptophan supplementation is a good therapy for patients with seasonal affective disorder.

"Patients with seasonal affective disorder (SAD) do not necessarily experience depressive episodes every winter. We assessed whether the behavioural response to tryptophan depletion in summer when patients are fully remitted and off therapy is capable of predicting a future depressive episode of SAD. In a prospective study design, we followed up 11 consenting SAD patients who had undergone tryptophan depletion during summer. We evaluated how many of these patients would develop a depressive episode in the subsequent fall/winter. Seven out of eight patients who relapsed during tryptophan depletion in summer developed a depressive episode in the subsequent winter. Two out of the three patients who did not relapse during tryptophan depletion remained well during the follow-up period. Our preliminary findings suggest that those SAD patients who develop depressive symptoms during tryptophan depletion when they are fully remitted and off therapy remain at high risk to experience a depressive episode of SAD also in the subsequent winter."[36]

Lam RW, et al[37], studied patients with seasonal affective disorder and found that many of them do not respond to light therapy, whereas, treatment with tryptophan was effective. This further supports previous discussions that low serotonin is the major cause of seasonal affective disorder and that tryptophan is a good therapy.

"OBJECTIVE: Up to one-third of patients with seasonal affective disorder (SAD) do not have a full response to light therapy. Given the evidence for serotonergic dysregulation in SAD, we examined the possible role of l-tryptophan as an augmentation strategy for nonresponders and partial responders to light therapy. METHOD: Eligible drug-free patients meeting DSM-IV criteria for SAD were treated for 2 weeks using a standard morning light therapy regimen (10,000 lux cool-white fluorescent light for 30 minutes). Partial and nonresponders were treated for 2 weeks with open-label l-tryptophan (1 g 3 times daily) while light therapy was continued. Ratings at baseline and follow-up included the 29-item Structured Interview Guide for the Hamilton Depression Rating Scale, SAD version (SIGH-SAD) and the Clinical Global Impression (CGI) scale. RESULTS: Sixteen patients began the l-tryptophan augmentation phase. Two patients discontinued medications within 3 days because of side effects. In the 14 patients completing treatment, the addition of l-tryptophan resulted in significant reduction of mean depression scores. Nine of 14 patients

(64%) showed very good clinical responses to combined treatment and minimal side effects. CONCLUSION: This open-label study suggests that l-tryptophan may be an effective augmentation strategy for those patients with SAD who show limited or poor response to bright light therapy. Further placebo-controlled studies are warranted to demonstrate efficacy."[37]

Causes of Serotonin and Norepinephrine Imbalance

Insufficiency of Related Chemicals to Produce Serotonin and Norepinephrine

Figure 1 – Serotonin Pathways and Figure 2 – Catecholamine Pathways, illustrate the biochemical pathways that produce serotonin and norepinephrine using various amino acids, vitamins, minerals, and enzymes. A deficiency of any of these chemicals will stop the production of the associated neurotransmitters.

Chemical Depletion of Serotonin and Norepinephrine

There are a number of chemicals which cause the destruction of neurotransmitters in the synaptic junction including monamine oxidase that metabolizes neurotransmitters naturally after they have been used to transmit signals. Neurotoxic chemicals such as hydrocarbons and pesticides cause the destruction of neurotransmitters before they are used to transmit signals. Tyramine is a commonly found chemical that displaces serotonin and norepinephrine before it has been used to transmit signals. Tyramine will be explained further in the next section.

The chemical reserpine found in red wine depletes norepinephrine and serotonin. Any fermented product will contain tyramine, which displaces norepinephrine directly and serotonin indirectly through increased vasoconstriction, which eventually depletes serotonin.

> "There was a high correlation ($r = 0.87$) between the effect of red wine and that of reserpine in different individuals. Some types of red wine caused a consistently higher release of 5-HT than others in all subjects; one red wine in particular resulted in negligible release. Preliminary studies, using solid phase

extraction methods, showed that the active components lie mainly in a subgroup of the flavonoid fraction."[38]

S.Y. YEH, et al[39], investigated the mechanisms of serotonin depletion after the use of antihistamines. This study demonstrates one of many ways in which serotonin is depleted in serotonin related disorders.

"This study investigated the effects of chlorpheniramine (CPA, 10–25 mg/kg), diphenhydramine (DIPH, 20 mg/kg), tripelennamine (TRIP, 20 mg/kg), and pyrilamine (PYRI, 20 mg/kg) on 3,4-methylenedioxymethamphetamine (MDMA, 20 mg/kg). MDMA increased body temperature and decreased levels of indoles, measured by HPLC, in several brain regions of rats. Possible mechanisms of the different effects of the antihistamines on MDMA-induced hyperthermia and depletion of serotonin are discussed."[39]

Neurotoxic chemicals are a major problem in depleting neurotransmitters. In the study by Kanada M, et al[40], that neurotoxic chemicals lowered the levels of serotonin, dopamine, norepinephrine in the brain. They also found that the turnover rates of serotonin and norepinephrine were increased. The faster the turnover rate, the faster the depletion of neurotransmitters if they are replaced at least at the same rate by which they are depleted. The study also found the levels of acetylcholine in the brain to be increased. Acetylcholine is a neurotransmitter that causes excitatory actions, which probably is responsible for the increased turnover rates of serotonin and norepinephrine.

"We investigated the effects of oral administration of 28 organic chemical agents, all of which possess neurotoxicity and most of which are used as industrial solvents, on monoamine neurotransmitters and metabolites in the rat brain. Each chemical was administered to rats singly at a dose of one-quarter the LD50 value. Two hours after administration, acetylcholine, 3,4-dihydroxyphenylalanine (DOPA), dopamine, 3,4-dihydroxyphenylacetic acid (DOPAC), homovanillic acid (HVA), norepinephrine, 3-methoxy-4-hydroxyphenylglycol (MHPG), serotonin, and 5-hydroxyindoleacetic acid (5HIAA) contents in the small-brain regions were measured. Twenty-one of the 28 chemicals increased acetylcholine in the hippocampus, a ratio (21/28) far higher than the 0.5 expected were these chemicals to have no tendency to increase or decrease acetylcholine. This ratio was calculated for each brain substance. Large differences from

0.5 were also obtained for DOPAC (higher), and for 5HIAA and three neurotransmitters (dopamine, norepinephrine, and serotonin) in the hypothalamus (all lower). The ratios for MHPG and 5HIAA in the medulla oblongata were very high. In the hypothalamus, the concentrations of brain substances were easily altered by the test chemicals, and the turnover rates of hypothalamic norepinephrine and serotonin in the medulla oblongata seemed to be accelerated."[40]

Tyramine Depletion of Serotonin and Norepinephrine

Tyramine displaces norepinephrine from sympathetic nerve endings and epinephrine from the adrenal glands. Initially, this release results in increased sympathetic stimulation, which causes higher blood pressure, insomnia, increased aggression in some cases, increased glucose release, increased metabolism, inhibition of the G.I. tract, and increased cardiovascular activity. Increased sympathetic stimulation can also result in a depletion of serotonin. The final result is a depletion of norepinephrine, epinephrine, and serotonin reserves. An individual's activity, as a result of tyramine intake, may initially go from mania to depression and migraine headaches later on. The presence of monoamine oxidase in the gastrointestinal tract will inactivate tyramine.

Why does tyramine affect some people and not others? The level of monoamine oxidase in the gut varies from person to person. If there is more tyramine in the gut than the amount of monoamine oxidase that is needed to break it down, tyramine will get into the blood stream.

Compounds with tyraminase properties will be helpful in the treatment of lost serotonin and norepinephrine after tyramine ingestion. So far, none have been found.

The tyramine content in foods varies greatly due to different processing, aging, fermentation, ripening and/or contamination. Many foods that contain small amounts of tyramine develop large amounts of tyramine if the food products were left to spoil, age (not fresh), or ferment. The emphasis is placed on FRESH FOODS. Fruits that are permissible should be very fresh. Avoid leftovers kept in the refrigerator especially meats, dry packages mixes, canned products (prepared foods), yeast extracts, and protein extracts. Remember, foods increase in their tyramine content as they age or ferment. For example, bananas are permissible if they are fresh, not if they are overripe.

Tyramine can also be produced by bacteria in the gastrointestinal track. Helicobacter pylori can produce large amounts of tyramine in the gut. Various bacteria, including probiotics in the gut can cause an increase in the production of tyramine.

The brain converts tryptophan to serotonin. Serotonin itself cannot transport into the brain, it needs to be manufactured there. Tryptophan requires an albumin carrier to transport into the brain. Tryptophan competes with amino acids and fatty acids to attach to the albumin carrier. High carbohydrates will increase the body's ability to transport tryptophan into the brain. So, when the brain is low in serotonin, it creates an appetite for carbohydrates.

Mild tyramine reactions can occur almost immediately after the ingestion of approximately 6 mg of tyramine in a single portion. Severe reactions can occur almost immediately after the ingestion 10-25 mg of tyramine. Blood pressure will begin to rise within several hours after ingestion of tyramine.

Approximate tyramine contents of food[15]:
Cheddar cheese = 1.5 mg/g (42.5 mg/ounce)
Blue Stilton = 0.2 mg/g (5.6 mg/ounce)
Gouda = 0.02 mg/g (0.56 mg/ounce)
Beer = 0.02 mg/g (0.56 mg/ounce)
Wine = 0.025 mg/g (0.71 mg/ounce)
Yeast Extracts = 2 mg/g (56.6 mg/ounce)

"It was found that some cheeses contain high concentrations of tyramine. This amine causes intense pressor responses in man because it releases norepinephrine."[41]

Figure 6 – Tyramine Pathways

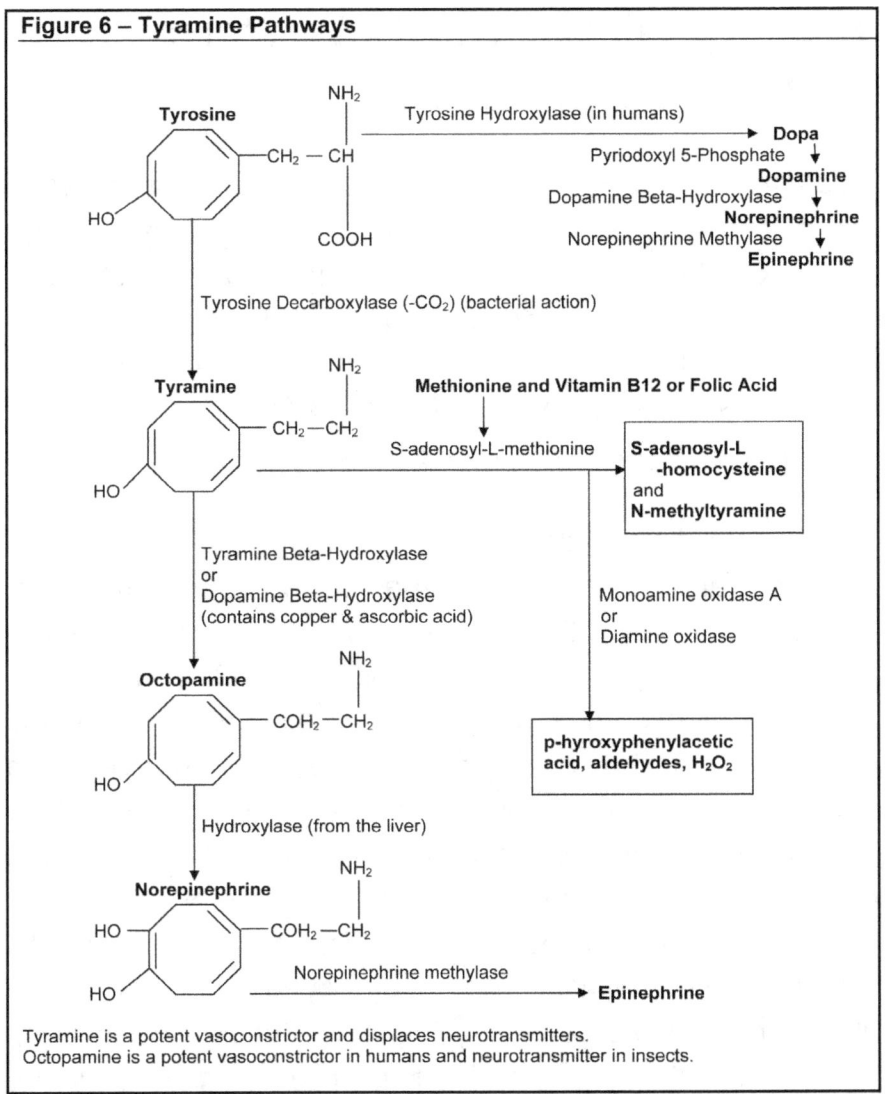

Tyramine is a potent vasoconstrictor and displaces neurotransmitters.
Octopamine is a potent vasoconstrictor in humans and neurotransmitter in insects.

Figure 6 – Tyramine Pathways, illustrates how tyrosine is broken down into tyramine by bacteria. This is also the fermentation process used to make yogurt, cheeses, etc.

77

Inflammatory Eicosanoid Serotonin Depletion

Eicosanoids (eye–cos-an-oids) are chemical messengers in two different forms, pro-inflammatory and anti-inflammatory. The pro-inflammatory variety stimulate vasoconstriction, platelet aggregation, tissue repair, clot formation, allergic responses, renin secretion, increased glycogenolysis, immune suppression, insulin release inhibition, and norepinephrine release inhibition.

Arachidonic acid, after being activated by the enzyme cyclooxygenase, produces the series 2 eicosanoids, prostaglandin-2 and thromboxane. Series 2 eicosanoids are pro-inflammatory, vasoconstrictive, platelet aggregating, allergic response stimulating, etc. Arachidonic acid after the activation of the enzyme lipoxygenase, converts to hydroperoxyeicosatetraenoic acid and leukotrienes. These eicosanoids are also pro-inflammatory, etc. Leukotrienes are more potent than prostaglandins and thromboxanes and much more inflammatory than histamine. Leukotrienes cause vasoconstriction, platelet aggregation, and stimulate allergic response creating a positive feedback to sustain the allergic reactions already in progress. As discussed previously, vasoconstriction causes the loss of serotonin by accelerating its use. They also suppress immune function, and constrict airways which can elevate carbon dioxide levels in the blood. Serotonin and histamine are released when basophil cells burst and excreted into the urine.

Eicosapentanoic Acid (EPA) and Docosahexanoic Acid (DHA) produce the series 3 eicosanoids and prostaglandin-3. The series 3 eicosanoids are anti-inflammatory like the series 1 eicosanoids. EPA and DHA also displace arachidonic acid, reducing the demand for cholesterol synthesis, stimulates metabolism of fat stores, activates t-lymphocytes, and enhances action of insulin. Series 3 eicosanoids are found to be low in diabetes, coronary heart disease, depressives, and alcoholics.

When tryptophan or 5-HTP enters the body, when the body is low in serotonin, the tryptophan or 5-HTP will be used by the body first. If there is any tryptophan or 5-HTP remaining, they will be available to the brain.

In conclusion, red meat and foods containing arachidonic acid should be avoided in order to avoid inflammatory reactions whereby serotonin is lost. Furthermore, eicosapentanoic acid and docosahexanoic acid (omega 3 fatty acids) should be taken to counteract inflammatory reactions.

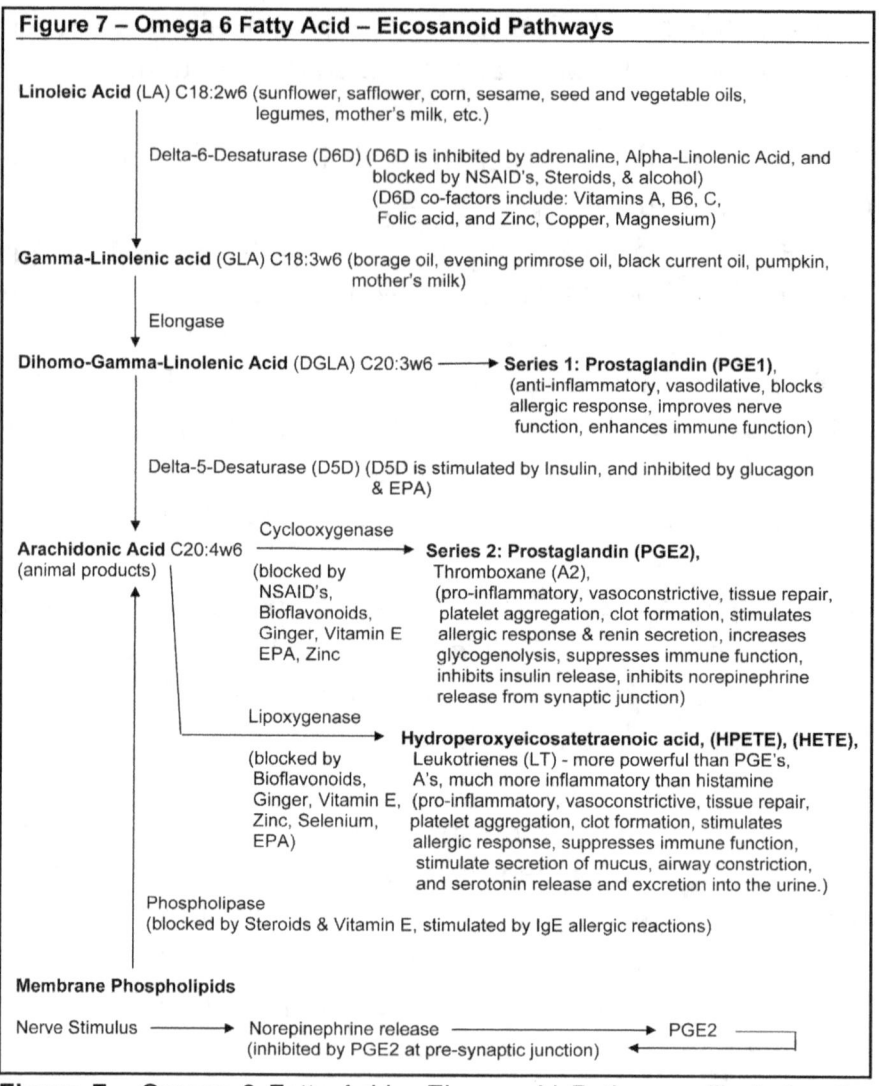

Figure 7 – Omega 6 Fatty Acid – Eicosanoid Pathways

Linoleic Acid (LA) C18:2w6 (sunflower, safflower, corn, sesame, seed and vegetable oils, legumes, mother's milk, etc.)

Delta-6-Desaturase (D6D) (D6D is inhibited by adrenaline, Alpha-Linolenic Acid, and blocked by NSAID's, Steroids, & alcohol)
(D6D co-factors include: Vitamins A, B6, C, Folic acid, and Zinc, Copper, Magnesium)

Gamma-Linolenic acid (GLA) C18:3w6 (borage oil, evening primrose oil, black current oil, pumpkin, mother's milk)

Elongase

Dihomo-Gamma-Linolenic Acid (DGLA) C20:3w6 ⟶ **Series 1: Prostaglandin (PGE1),**
(anti-inflammatory, vasodilative, blocks allergic response, improves nerve function, enhances immune function)

Delta-5-Desaturase (D5D) (D5D is stimulated by Insulin, and inhibited by glucagon & EPA)

Cyclooxygenase
Arachidonic Acid C20:4w6 ⟶ **Series 2: Prostaglandin (PGE2),**
(animal products)   (blocked by   Thromboxane (A2),
                            NSAID's,   (pro-inflammatory, vasoconstrictive, tissue repair,
                            Bioflavonoids,   platelet aggregation, clot formation, stimulates
                            Ginger, Vitamin E allergic response & renin secretion, increases
                            EPA, Zinc   glycogenolysis, suppresses immune function,
                                             inhibits insulin release, inhibits norepinephrine
                                             release from synaptic junction)

Lipoxygenase
                            Hydroperoxyeicosatetraenoic acid, (HPETE), (HETE),
(blocked by   Leukotrienes (LT) - more powerful than PGE's,
Bioflavonoids,   A's, much more inflammatory than histamine
Ginger, Vitamin E,   (pro-inflammatory, vasoconstrictive, tissue repair,
Zinc, Selenium,   platelet aggregation, clot formation, stimulates
EPA)   allergic response, suppresses immune function,
                            stimulate secretion of mucus, airway constriction,
                            and serotonin release and excretion into the urine.)

Phospholipase
(blocked by Steroids & Vitamin E, stimulated by IgE allergic reactions)

Membrane Phospholipids

Nerve Stimulus ⟶ Norepinephrine release ⟶ PGE2
(inhibited by PGE2 at pre-synaptic junction)

Figure 7 - Omega 6 Fatty Acid - Eicosanoid Pathways, illustrates the various enzymes that control the inflammatory and anti-inflammatory processes.

80

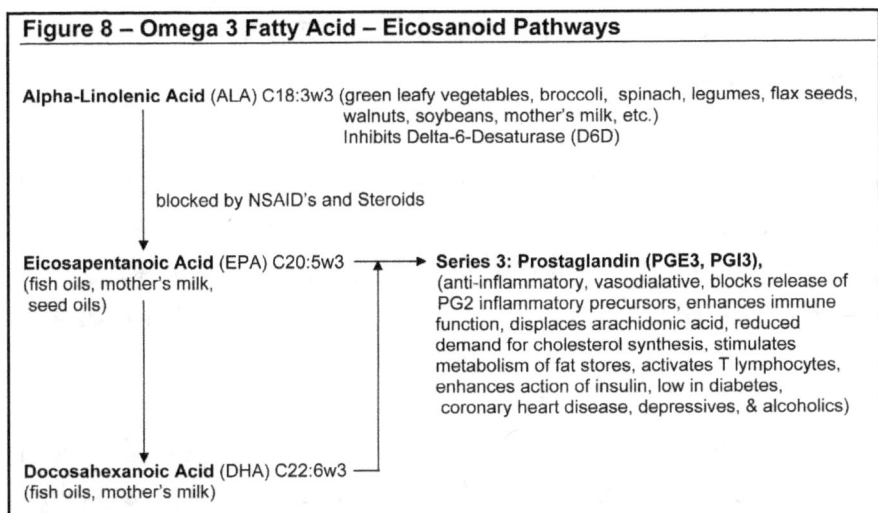

Figure 8 – Omega 3 Fatty Acid – Eicosanoid Pathways

Alpha-Linolenic Acid (ALA) C18:3w3 (green leafy vegetables, broccoli, spinach, legumes, flax seeds, walnuts, soybeans, mother's milk, etc.)
Inhibits Delta-6-Desaturase (D6D)

blocked by NSAID's and Steroids

Eicosapentanoic Acid (EPA) C20:5w3 ———▶ **Series 3: Prostaglandin (PGE3, PGI3),**
(fish oils, mother's milk,   (anti-inflammatory, vasodialative, blocks release of
 seed oils)   PG2 inflammatory precursors, enhances immune
        function, displaces arachidonic acid, reduced
        demand for cholesterol synthesis, stimulates
        metabolism of fat stores, activates T lymphocytes,
        enhances action of insulin, low in diabetes,
        coronary heart disease, depressives, & alcoholics)

Docosahexanoic Acid (DHA) C22:6w3 ———
(fish oils, mother's milk)

Figure 8 - Omega 3 Fatty Acid - Eicosanoid Pathways illustrates the use of eicosapentanoic acid and docosahexanoic acid in reducing inflammation.

Allergic Reactions and Serotonin Depletion

Allergic tendency is a phenomenon that is passed on genetically and characterized by large quantities of antibodies called reagins or sensitizing antibodies. When the allergen enters the body, the result is an allergen-reagin reaction.

Allergic reactions can cause the loss of serotonin when basophil cells rupture. IgE, IgM, and IgG antibodies which are immunoglobin reagins or sensitizing antibodies are generally passed on from parent to child. IgE, IgM, and IgG antibodies have an affinity to become attached to basophils and mast cells. When a specific antigen reacts with the antibody, the resulting attachment of the antigen to the antibody causes the basophil and/or mast cell to rupture, releasing large quantities of bradycin, histamine, serotonin, lysosomal enzymes, and activates phospholipases, which are usually excreted into the urine.

Emotional Stress, Alcohol, and Serotonin Depletion

As illustrated in Figure 1 – Serotonin Pathways, emotional stress and alcohol activate the enzyme tryptophan oxygenase, which causes tryptophan to be converted into kynurenine, nicotinic acid, picolinic acid, and acetyl CoA, instead of serotonin. Therefore, there will be less tryptophan available to the brain to make serotonin.

LeMarquand D, et al[42] have shown that there is a depletion of serotonin with alcohol use. Studies have also investigated violence and alcohol. The reason that some people become violent on alcohol may be due to a norepinephrine and epinephrine increase.

> "It is concluded that serotonin mediates ethanol intake as a part of its larger role in behavior modulation, such that increases in serotonergic functioning decrease ethanol intake, and decreased serotonergic functioning increases ethanol intake. Ethanol produces transient increases in serotonergic functioning that activate the mesolimbic dopaminergic reward system. The results are discussed in light of recent theories describing the regulatory role of serotonin in general behavior."[42]

Coincidentally, the emotional center of the brain (the limbic system) is also the part of the brain that controls bodily functions. The limbic system primarily includes the hypothalamus, the hippocampus, and the amygdala. The limbic system plays a key role in an individual's emotional life and with the formation of memories. As discussed previously, the amygdala is responsible for moral behavior. Emotional stress leads to undesirable nervous system reactions, hormonal reactions and biochemical pathway changes throughout the body. Continuous emotional stress will have adverse effects on every cell in the body with adverse effects of long-term hormonal, leukotriene, thromboxane, and inflammatory prostaglandin production. Emotional stress, alcohol, and a tryptophan dose greater than two grams, will activate the enzyme tryptophan oxygenase, which converts tryptophan into kynurenine, which then undergoes several conversions to become nicotinic acid (niacin), picolinic acid, and acetyl CoA. By converting much of the tryptophan into niacin and other compounds, there is less tryptophan available to be converted into serotonin. Tryptophan has to be administered in doses less than two grams to avoid the loss of tryptophan to its conversion to kynurenine.

Emotional stress causes an increase in epinephrine in the fight or flight response, which in turn converts norepinephrine into epinephrine, depleting the norepinephrine reserves. An increase in norepinephrine and epinephrine leads to vasoconstriction and the eventual depletion of serotonin reserves.

Emotional stress causes an increase in epinephrine in the fight or flight response, which in turn decreases the conversion of linoleic acid into gamma-lineolenic acid, thereby producing less anti-inflammatory prostaglandins. Inflammation can lead to serotonin depletion as previously discussed.

Changes in Gonadatropin Hormone Levels and Serotonin Levels

A study by Kugaya A, et al, demonstrated an increase in prefrontal serotonin receptors following estrogen administration.[44] Chouinard et al., 1987, found that estrogen lifts the mood and when combined with progesterone, stabilizes bipolar mood swings. Estrogen appears to enhance serotonin levels. However, low estrogen has the opposite effect. High amounts of estrogen can induce a multitude of metabolic disturbances. Progesterone's primary influence on serotonin metabolism is in counterbalancing estrogen.

> 5-HT(2A) receptor binding was significantly increased after estrogen replacement therapy in the right prefrontal cortex (right precentral gyrus [Brodmann's area 9], inferior frontal gyrus [Brodmann's area 47], medial frontal gyrus [Brodmann's area 6, 10] and the anterior cingulate cortex [Brodmann's area 32]). CONCLUSIONS: Estrogen increases 5-HT(2A) receptor binding in human prefrontal regions.[44]

Studies[45] link high levels of the male hormone testosterone to aggression. However, elevated testosterone alone doesn't account for aggressive behavior. Athletes and businessmen tend to have high testosterone levels, without being any more violence or prone to violence than people with low testosterone. Paul C. Bernhardt[45] suggests that testosterone may not act alone in promoting aggression. Rather, he suggests, aggressive men's behavior may be influenced by high testosterone levels combined with low levels of the brain chemical serotonin. Bernhardt speculates that the hypothalamus and amygdala, "prominently associated with both testosterone and serotonin," play a key role in aggressive responses to situations in which efforts at dominance are frustrated. He notes that low serotonin levels have been found in the hypothalamus and the amygdala in aggressive animals," and that testosterone action in both of these brain structures has been shown to increase aggression.

There is a great difference between aggression and violence. Aggression may be considered as enthusiastically promoting an idea of some kind the way salespeople do. Violence may be considered as behavior ranging from yelling to physically attacking another person.

Intestinal Dysbiosis and Serotonin Depletion

Candida Albicans (Yeast) infections are a common problem. Continuing research on intestinal Candida Albicans overgrowth indicates that our lifestyles with diets high in sugars, widespread use of antibiotics (much of which is passed on to humans from the meat of farm animals that have been fed antibiotics), environmental pollution, stress, steroid drugs, and birth control pills along with the lack of acidophilus and bifidobacteria supplementation carries a lot of the blame for this persistent and growing health concern. Clinical Symptoms include: abdominal bloating, intestinal gas, Indigestion, constipation or diarrhea, chemical sensitivities, food allergies, hypoglycemia, premenstrual tension, endometriosis, prostatitis, vaginitis, chronic dermatological infections or rashes, acne, inability to concentrate, frequent mood shifts, loss of memory fatigue/ lethargy, depression, desire for refined carbohydrates or yeast containing foods.

Various toxins are produced by bacteria and yeast. Intestinal bacteria produce a significant amount of ammonia[47]. Too much ammonia increases the turnover of serotonin in the brain and interferes with mitochondrial energy production. Ammonia will also increase GABA[48], an inhibitory neurotransmitter in the central nervous system, changing the way other neurotransmitters are used. A large number of toxins, including aflatoxin, acetaldehyde (similar to formaldehyde), and gliotoxin, have been identified coming from yeast, including Candida Albicans. Acetaldehyde reduces the ability of red blood cells to accept, hold, and transport oxygen through the bloodstream. Acetaldehyde induces a deficiency of vitamin B1 (thiamin), niacin, Pyridoxal-5-Phosphate. Acetaldehyde reduces Acetyl Coenzyme A and impairs cellular energy production. Acetaldehyde unfavorably influences prostaglandin metabolism. Acetaldehyde may alter normal brain function due to its tendency to combine in the brain with two key neurotransmitters, dopamine and serotonin. Molybdenum is helpful in breaking down Acetaldehyde.

> "Acetaldehyde is a particularly toxic substance which, in addition to being produced from threonine and ethanol, it is a product of the metabolism (i.e. fermentation) of carbohydrate in yeast hence, the Candida connection. Acetaldehyde is thought to be the major source of tissue damage in alcoholics rather than ethanol itself."[49]

Intestinal Candida Albicans overgrowth, as the result of antibiotic therapy, is associated with intestinal overgrowth of the bacteria Clostridium difficile[15]. There are also many bacteria that enter the stomach from the food supply. If an individual is experiencing stress, that individual may not produce enough hydrochloric acid to destroy microorganisms that enter the stomach from food. Helicobacter pylori are typical bacteria that invade the stomach and may eventually cause ulceration in the stomach or intestinal lining. Clostridia bacteria produce dihydroxyphenylpyruvic acid (DHPPA)[49], a molecular mimic of norepinephrine and dopamine. The symptoms of Clostridium difficile overgrowth are similar to that of Candida Albicans overgrowth, and may include ulcerative colitis, anemia, and malabsorption. Ulcerative colitis can lead to weight loss. Malabsorption can lead to excessive eating and weight gain.

Increased intestinal permeability (leaky gut) is a major cause of food intolerance, sensitivity, and allergy[15]. The small intestine is an organ that absorbs nutrients and acts as a barrier to toxic compounds and large molecules. Increased intestinal permeability is referred to as "leaky gut syndrome," which allows toxic compounds and large molecules to enter the lymphatic and blood system including neurotoxins that deplete serotonin and norepinephrine. Increased intestinal permeability can be caused by: Candida Albicans overgrowth, non-steroidal anti-inflammatory drugs (NSAID's), HIV infection, intestinal infection, intestinal dysboisis, maldigestion, malabsorption, alcoholism, aging, deficient IgA, giardiasis, candidiasis, ingestion of allergic foods, ingestion of offending chemicals, and trauma and endotoxima.

Often the bowel is ignored as being associated with health disorders. Constipation is such a widespread problem that laxatives are one of the highest selling classes of drugs in this country. Imagine food sitting on a table decaying for weeks, months and even years. What will happen if this food is eaten? This is analogous to food that remains in the large intestines for the same length of time. Many of the decayed materials and toxins get into the blood stream and have an adverse effect on health. Bacterial action plays a major role in nutrition and digestion. Friendly bacteria synthesize valuable nutrients by digesting portions of the fecal mass. Vitamin K, portions of the B-complex, and other vitamins are produced by bacteria. Any remaining proteins are broken down by the bacterial and fungal flora. Other bacterial byproducts include: indole, skatole, hydrogen sulfide, fatty acids, methane gas, and carbon dioxide. The normal bacterial flora can easily be destroyed by antibiotics. Destruction of the bacterial flora in the intestinal tract can lead to the overgrowth of Candida albicans and Clostridium difficile in the intestines. The results are malabsorption of vitamins and the production of neurotoxins. An individual may move their bowels regularly, but may have material covering the lining of the colon (like a partially clogged water pipe).

Dehydration

There is a great tendency for many people to dehydrate from not drinking enough water. The mechanism the body uses for eliminating toxins is to convert them from fat-soluble to water-soluble so they can be excreted by the kidneys, bowels, and skin. Dehydration can cause a build up of toxins, particularly neurotoxins that deplete serotonin and norepinephrine. Drinking plenty of pure water will allow the body to rapidly excrete soluble toxins. Water is also important because it moves material along the intestinal tract. For most people, drink a minimum of 2 quarts of water per day. Water deprivation is associated with depletion of serotonin, which is characterized by an increase in the serotonin metabolite 5-HIAA.[43]

> "Water deprivation was associated with a significant increase in 5-HIAA levels in the midbrain and hypothalamus, along with a decrease in serotonin levels and a three-fold increase in serotonin catabolism (the 5-HIAA:serotonin concentration ratio). Hyperhydration induced moderate increases in serotonin and 5-HIAA levels in the hypothalamus with no changes in the midbrain. The blood corticosterone level doubled in water deprivation and decreased in hyperhydration. It is suggested that activation of the

serotoninergic system induces a complex adaptive reaction in water deprivation, including mechanisms specific for the regulation of water-electrolyte homeostasis and non-specific stress mechanisms (vasopressin and corticoliberin secretion)."[43]

The hydration calculator below will help to determine the correct amount of water for an individual. It is obvious a five-foot, 100 pound woman doesn't require the same amount of water that a seven-foot, 300 pound man does.

Hydration Calculator

Multiply weight in pounds by   0.5   _____

Multiply minutes of exercise per day by   0.1   _____

If pregnant, add   16   _____

If breast feeding, add   24   _____

If in a high altitude, add   8   _____

If in a dry climate, add   8   _____

Multiply number of caffeinated drinks per day by 4   _____

Multiply number of alcoholic drinks per day by   8   _____

If the weather very hot or very cold, add   16   _____

If there is fever or diarrhea, add   8   _____

Ounces of water needed per day, add totals   _____

Quarts of water needed per day, divide totals by 32   _____

8 oz. glasses of water needed per day, divide totals by 8 _____

Hydration Calculator References: Mayo Clinic, International Bottled Water Association, The United States Army Research Institute of Environmental Medicine, Centers for Disease Control, Water for Good Health

High Glycemic Diet

The endocrine system and the nervous system work together to regulate the appetite so that the correct amount and the correct kind of food is taken in. Refined white sugar and starches have a high glycemic index that offsets this balance. This high-caloric dynamite drives the pancreas and pituitary gland into hyper-secretion of hormones and enzymes, especially insulin. Eating added sugar in various foods and drinks everyday chronically over-stimulates the pituitary and pancreas glands. The thyroid and adrenals also suffer. Many medical journals have implicated refined white sugar as a causative factor in: arteriosclerosis, coronary heart disease, kidney disease, liver disease, shortening of life span, making blood platelets stick together, causing rise in serum triglycerides and cholesterol, and increasing the desire for coffee and tobacco. Studies have shown that lower insulin levels promote rapid fat loss, increased energy level, lower blood pressure, and lower cholesterol. The increase in insulin activates the enzyme Delta5-Desaturase, which converts arachidonic acid into inflammatory eicosanoids, which lead to the decrease of serotonin and norepinephrine as previously described.

The glycemic index is a relative scale for classifying foods according to the blood sugar response that they cause. It measures how fast the carbohydrate of a particular food is converted to glucose and enters the blood. The glycemic index for a particular food may be different for different individuals and at different ages.

Why is this important? When glucose enters the blood, insulin is produced by the pancreas into the blood stream. Insulin enters the cells and facilitates the transport of glucose into the cells for energy, storage, and maintenance. Insulin also helps to transport other nutrients into the cells such as vitamins, minerals, amino acids and fatty acids. The amount of insulin produced is proportional to the amount of glucose in the blood at a particular time.

Insulin increases the activity of a liver enzyme called HMG CoA reductase, which causes the liver to produce more cholesterol. Insulin stimulates trigylceride production. Insulin also increases the activity of an enzyme called delta 5 desaturase, which converts dihomogammalinolenic acid to arachidonic acid, which produces vasoconstrictors and inflammatory eicosanoids, which stimulates allergic reactions and decrease immune function.

Foods that contain higher amounts of fiber, fat, and protein will have a lower glycemic Index. Fiber, fat, and protein slows the uptake of sugar into the blood stream. Foods that have a high glycemic index will be broken down into glucose faster and therefore enter the blood stream faster, hence causing more insulin to be produced.

The glycemic index is a relative scale for classifying foods according to the blood sugar response that they cause. It measures how fast the carbohydrate of a particular food is converted to glucose and enters the blood. The glycemic index for a particular food may be different for different individuals. The figures below contain the glycemic index values for the average individual.

The numbers used in the glycemic index are percentages with respect to a reference food. In this list, they are given with respect to glucose. For example, brown rice, which has a glycemic index of 58, raises blood sugar more than barley, which has a glycemic index of 26. A food is generally considered to have a high Glycemic Index if it is greater than 50 (1/2 of the value of glucose), which is indicated by the "High-Low Point" in the table below. Glycemic Index values of foods below are adjusted proportionately so that Glycemic Index of glucose is equal to 100.

Avoid eating sugar (sucrose) from this point forward. Fructose (the sugar in fruit) is an excellent substitute. Sugar (sucrose) has a glycemic index of 67. Fructose has a glycemic index of 23. Fructose is technically one-third the glycemic index of sucrose. However, since fructose is twice as sweet to the taste as sucrose, you will use half as much. The effective glycemic index of fructose becomes one-sixth that of sucrose. Also note that protein enriched pasta has a glycemic index of about half that of white pasta. Many pastas are labeled as "enriched" but not "protein enriched," which may relate to iron enriched not protein enriched – read the labels carefully.

Glycemic Index

The following list is a compilation of Glycemic Index derived from several studies. The dashed line separates above and below 50.

Bakery Products
Cake, sponge --48
Cake, banana, made with sugar -----------------------49

Cake, pound --56
Pizza, cheese --63
Muffins --64
Cake, flan --68
Cake, angel food --69
Croissant--70
Crumpet--72
Donut--79
Waffles---80

Beverages
Coffee and Tea ---0
Soy milk --31

Soft drink, Fanta --71
Rice milk --85
Lucozade--99

Breads

Bürgen Soy Lin --20
Bürgen Oat Bran & Honey Loaf ------------------------------31
Barley kernel bread --40
Rye Kernel bread ---48
Fruit loaf--49
Oat bran bread --50
Mixed grain bread --50

Pumpernickel ---52
Bulger bread ---55
Linseed rye bread --57
Pita bread, white ---60
Whole grain bread ---65
Rye flour bread ---67
Semolina bread ---67
Oat kernel bread ---68
Barley flour bread--69
Wheat bread, wholemeal flour--------------------------72
Melba toast --73
Wheat bread, white---74
Bagel, white ---75
Wheat bread, gluten free ------------------------------94
French baguette--99

Breakfast Cereals

Rice Bran ---20
All-bran ---44

Cereal Grains

Cookies

Crackers

High Fibre Rye Crispread--------------------------------68
Breton Wheat Crackers --------------------------------70
Stoned Wheat Thins --------------------------------70
Water Crackers--------------------------------74
Rice Cakes --------------------------------80
Puffed Crispbread --------------------------------85

Dairy Foods

Cream --------------------------------0
Yogurt, low fat, artificially sweet --------------------------------15
Milk --------------------------------30
Yogurt, low fat, fruit sugar sweet --------------------------------34
Milk, chocolate, sugar sweetened --------------------------------36

Ice Cream--------------------------------64

Flours

Almond Flour--------------------------------15?
Soy Flour--------------------------------25
Rye Flour--------------------------------45
Quinoa Flour --------------------------------45
Kamut Flour --------------------------------45

Chestnut Flour--------------------------------65
Potato Starch --------------------------------95
White Rice Rlour --------------------------------95
Arrow Root Starch --------------------------------85

Fruit

Legumes

Broad beans (fava beans) --------------------------------82

Nuts/Seeds

Almonds ---15
Hazel nuts ---15
Cashew nuts --15
Walnuts---15
Sunflower seeds -------------------------------------35
Chestnut--60

Pasta

Spaghetti, protein enriched---------------------------28
Fettuccine--34
Vermicelli--37
Star pastina--39
Spaghetti, white -------------------------------------43
Linguine ---47
Instant noodles --------------------------------------49
Whole wheat --50

Spaghetti, durum-------------------------------------57
Lasagna (hard wheat) --------------------------------60
Couscous --68
Gnocchi--69
Lasagna (soft wheat) --------------------------------75
Rice pasta, brown -----------------------------------96

Rice

Root Vegetables

Snack Foods

Peanuts---15
Peanut button, unsweetened ---------------------------40

Jams and marmalades ----------------------------------51
Chocolate --51
Potato crisps ---56
Popcorn --58
Mars Bar ---66
Life Savers--73
Corn chips ---77
Jelly beans--83
Pretzels--85
Dates ---103

Soups

Tomato Soup---39
Lentil soup, canned ---46

Split pea soup --63
Black bean soup --67
Green pea soup, canned ----------------------------------69

Sugars/Sweeteners

Stevia ---0
Fructose (twice as sweet as sucrose) ----------------23
Lactose --47

Honey---61

High fructose corn syrup ---------------------------------65
Maple Syrup---65
Sucrose---67
Glucose--100
Maltodextrin---110
Maltose--110
Corn Syrup---115

Vegetables

Celery---15
Fennel --15
Mushrooms---15
Olives ---15
Lettuce--15
Spinach---15
Sprouted seeds --15
Eggplant--20
Peas, dried --23
Tomatoes---30
Turnip, raw---30
Peas, green --35
Marrowfat, dried---41
Peas, green --50

Sweet corn---65
Pumpkin---78
Turnip, cooked---85

Glycemic Index References

Frati-Munari, A.C. , The Glycemic Index of Some Foods Common in Mexico, Gac Med Mex, Vol. 127, No. 2, March-April 1991

Jenkins, David J.A. et al., Glycemic Index of Foods: a Physiological Basis for Carbohydrate Exchange; (The American Journal of Clinical

Jenkins, D.J.A. and Jenkins, A.L. Treatment of hypertriglceridemia and diabetes; (Journal of the American College of Nutrition.

Jenkins, David J.A. et al., Starchy Foods and Glycemic Index; Diabetes Care, Vol. 11, No. 2, February 1988.

Miller, Janette Brand, et al, Rice: a High or Low Glycemic Index Food?; The American Journal of Clinical Nutrition, Vol. 56, 1992.

Miller, Janette C. Brand., Importance of Glycemic Index in Diabetes; The American Journal of Clinical Nutrition, Vol. 59 (supplement), 1994.

Miller, Janette Brand, International tables of glycemic index; The American Journal of Clinical Nutrition, Vol. 62 (supplement), 1995.

Rassmussen, Ole., Day-to-day Variation of the Glycemic Response in Subjects with Insulin-dependent Diabetes with Standardized Premeal Blood Glucose and Prandial Insulin Concentrations; The American Journal of Clinical Nutrition, Vol. 57, 1993.

Smith, Ulf., Carbohydrates, Fat, and Insulin Action; The American Journal of Clinical Nutrition, Vol. 59 (supplement), 1994

Wolever, Thomas M.S. et al., The Glycemic Index: Methodology and Clinical Implications The American Journal of Clinical Nutrition, Vol. 54, 1991.

Wolever, Thomas M.S. et al., Glycemic Index of Fruits and Fruit Products in Patients with Diabetes; The International Journal of Food Sciences and Nutrition, Vol. 43, 1993.

www.montignac.com

Balancing Serotonin and Norepinephrine Levels Though Diet and Supplementation

Increase Neurotransmitter Production and Reduce Neurotransmitter Loss

Dr. Allocca's approach to balance the levels of serotonin and norepinephrine is to provide the brain with the ingredients it needs to make serotonin and norepinephrine through supplementation and prevent the loss of serotonin and norepinephrine through diet and supplementation.

Below is a list of items that need to be addressed in a comprehensive nutritional program to balance serotonin and norepinephrine.

1. Avoid the food on the "Avoid Food" list.

2. Eat low glycemic index foods.

3. Drink plenty of water.

4. Supplementation to provide the brain with the nutrients it needs to make serotonin and norepinephrine, decrease allergic reactions, and control glucose levels (Neurobiology Formula 12397)

5. Supplementation to control gonadatropin hormone levels in men and women over 40 (Progesterone, Pregnenolone, and DHEA).

6. Bowel cleansing and detoxification (cascara sagrada and activated charcoal). See Figure 9 – Detoxification Pathways.

7. Liver detoxification (silimaryn). See Figure 9 – Detoxification Pathways.

8. Destroy pathological microorganisms in the intestinal tract (oregano oil). A significant number of scientific studies have demonstrated the antimicrobial effects of Oregano oil.

9. Replenish lactobacillus bifidus intestinal flora (2 billion organisms, once a week maximum)

10. Additional nutrients to decrease seasonal allergic reactions (quercetin 300 mg additional 1-2x daily)

11. Additional nutrients to decrease inflammatory eicosanoids (EPA/DHA)

12. Melatonin to decrease serotonin load (melatonin 3 mg)

13. General health supplementation (multi vitamin and minderal, potassium citrate, and calcium citrate)

As seen in Figure 1 – Serotonin Pathways, 5-Hydroxytryptophan (5-HTP) is manufactured from Tryptophan by Ascorbic acid & Tryptophan Hydroxylase. Supplementation with 5-Hydroxytryptophan is preferred over tryptophan because 5-Hydroxytryptophan is a metabolite of tryptophan that does not require the albumin carrier to transport into the brain and 5-Hydroxytryptophan is clinically more effective. The chemical formula of 5-Hydroxytryptophan is $C_{11}H_{12}N_2O_3$. 5-Hydroxytryptophan is converted into serotonin (5-hydroxytryptamine or 5-HT) by L-amino-acid decarboxylase with the help of Vitamin B6.

Current research demonstrates the effectiveness of using 5-HTP for treating children with "night terrors," Fibromyalgia, sleep, depression, migraine, pain, and more. 5-HTP is also used as a supplement by users of MDMA (ecstasy) to help replenish depleted serotonin to alleviate some of the depression that sometimes occurs in the days following MDMA usage.

As illustrated in Figure 4 – Migraine Pathways and Figure 5 – Depression Pathways, there are a number of factors that can deplete serotonin and norepinephrine, which needs to be addressed in a comprehensive nutritional program.

As previously examined, balancing the level of norepinephrine is tricky. A practitioner needs to examine how much tyrosine and phenylalanine an individual is getting from food sources. Clinical observation and titration of tyrosine will be required to determine the proper dose of tyrosine for each individual. Additional tyrosine will probably not be required for individuals suffering with anxiety, stressful lifestyle, and bipolar syndrome, but will probably be required for individuals suffering from depression. To avoid promoting an increase of epinephrine, titration of tyrosine should be done carefully and with attention to the neurotransmitter dynamics.

Detoxification

Damage to the cells from toxins is the major cause of many health problems. Detoxifying and ridding the body of toxins, particularly neurotoxins, which deplete serotonin and norepinephrine, is an important part of balancing serotonin and norepinephrine levels.

Toxicity from foreign chemicals (exotoxins) can cause damage to almost all cells of the body. Symptoms include: fatigue, headaches, neurological disorders, chemical sensitivities, immune dysfunction, and liver disorders. Food is often the main source of toxins. There are thousands of chemicals used by the food industry during processing and packaging. Many farmers use pesticides on their produce, which are passed to consumers. In addition to these external sources of toxins, the body also produces toxins internally called, endotoxins resulting from digestion, immune system functions, emotional stress, etc. Endotoxins may also be produced as the result of food allergies and sensitivities.

Fat-soluble toxins are easily absorbed but poorly excreted. Often, they accumulate in the body causing damage to the tissues and organs, and depleting serotonin and norepinephrine. Fat-soluble chemicals are converted to water-soluble chemicals, primarily in the liver, and in some cells, in a two-step process so that the water-soluble toxins can be excreted by the urine, liver, and skin. The skin is a vitally important organ that eliminates toxins through perspiration.

During the first phase of detoxification, fat-soluble chemicals are converted into intermediate chemicals. As a result of this process, free radicals are produced. The free radicals and the intermediate chemicals can cause damage to the cells. An adequate amount of antioxidants must be present to detoxify these intermediate compounds produced during the first phase of detoxification. The first phase may also detoxify some chemicals directly without requiring a second phase conversion.

During the second phase, the intermediate chemicals are converted into water-soluble, chemicals, which are less toxic and easily excreted in the urine, bile, and skin.

It is very important to avoid toxic chemicals from the environment. Tap water should be filtered to remove lead, chlorine, heavy metals, and bacteria. It is also important to consume an adequate supply of anti-oxidants to prevention cellular damage.

The ability of the liver to detoxify is determined by the availability of the appropriate nutrients and enzymes. An adequate supply of antioxidants is vitally important after the first phase of converting fat-soluble toxins, which produce free radicals. Reduced glutathione, superoxide dismutase, and catalase are the primary antioxidants used in the body to neutralize free radicals. Other antioxidants include: beta-carotene, vitamin E, vitamin C, selenium, n-acetylcysteine, lipoic acid, and proanthocyanidins. Vitamin and mineral cofactors required for cytochrome P-450 reactions include: riboflavin, niacin, magnesium, iron, and other trace minerals. Phytochemicals such as indoles from cruciferous vegetables and quercetin also help during the first phase of detoxification. Other second phase conjugating agents include amino acids such as glycine, cysteine, glutamine, methionine, taurine, glutamic acid, and asparatic acid.

Vitamin, mineral, and protein deficiencies will decrease the activity of the detoxification pathways. Fats and polyunsaturated oils can promote the uptake of many chemical carcinogens in the gastrointestinal tract. Olive oil (monounsaturated) and omega 3 polyunsaturated oils (EPA, DHA) have a neutral effect in promoting the uptake of carcinogens in the gastrointestinal tract.

As previously discussed, the detoxification process requires various nutrients to function. Without such nutrients in the cells, intermediate compounds can cause cellular and DNA damage. If the apoptosis system (cells self destruct if they are damaged) does not get the proper nutrients, the damaged cells can reproduce. If the immune system does not get the proper nutrients, the damaged cells can reproduce out of control causing cancer.

Transporting the nutrients into the blood is only the first step. The nutrients must enter the cells in order to be available for use by the cells. In order for the nutrients to get into the cells, they must be transported though the cell membrane. When there is a lack of nutrients, particularly oxygen inside the cell, there is a build-up of lactic acid inside the cell. Excessive lactic acid damages the cell membrane transport mechanism and DNA. Lactic acid causes the cell to become acidic (lower pH). There is a correlation between intracellular pH and urine pH. The urine pH must be 6.5 or greater, which indicates the maximum amount of lactic acid in the cell, for the membrane transport mechanisms to function at peak performance.

The detoxification process requires various nutrients to function properly. Without such nutrients in the cells, intermediate compounds can cause cellular and DNA damage. If the apoptosis system (cells self destruct if they are damaged), does not get the proper nutrients, the damaged cells can reproduce. If the immune system does not get the proper nutrients, the damaged cells can reproduce out of control causing cancer.

Transporting the nutrients into the blood is only the first step. The nutrients must enter the cells in order to be available for use by the cells. Nutrients are transported though the cell membrane to the inside of the cell, were they are used to create energy in the form of ATP. When there is a lack of nutrients, particularly oxygen inside the cell, there is a build-up of lactic acid inside the cell. Excessive lactic acid, damages the cell membrane transport mechanism and DNA. Lactic acid causes the cell to become acidic (lower pH). There is a correlation between intracellular pH and urine/saliva pH. The urine/saliva pH must be 6.5 or greater for the membrane transport mechanisms to function.

The Ascorbate Flush

The ascorbate flush is used to increase body pH, cleanse the bowels, dilate the common (bile) duct while stimulating the liver to release toxins, and to determine the daily dose of Vitamin C. Mix 1/2 teaspoon of ascorbate powder with 2 ounces of room temperature water or juice. Allow the effervescence to dissipate (about 2 minutes), then drink the mixture. Repeat this procedure every 15 minutes until a watery diarrhea has occurred, while writing down the times and doses taken. After achieving the watery diarrhea, add up the total amount of ascorbate taken.

The daily amount will be 50 percent of the total (5,000 mg maximum). Each 1/2 teaspoon of vitamin C powder should be equal to 1,500 mg of vitamin C and contain magnesium, calcium, and potassium.

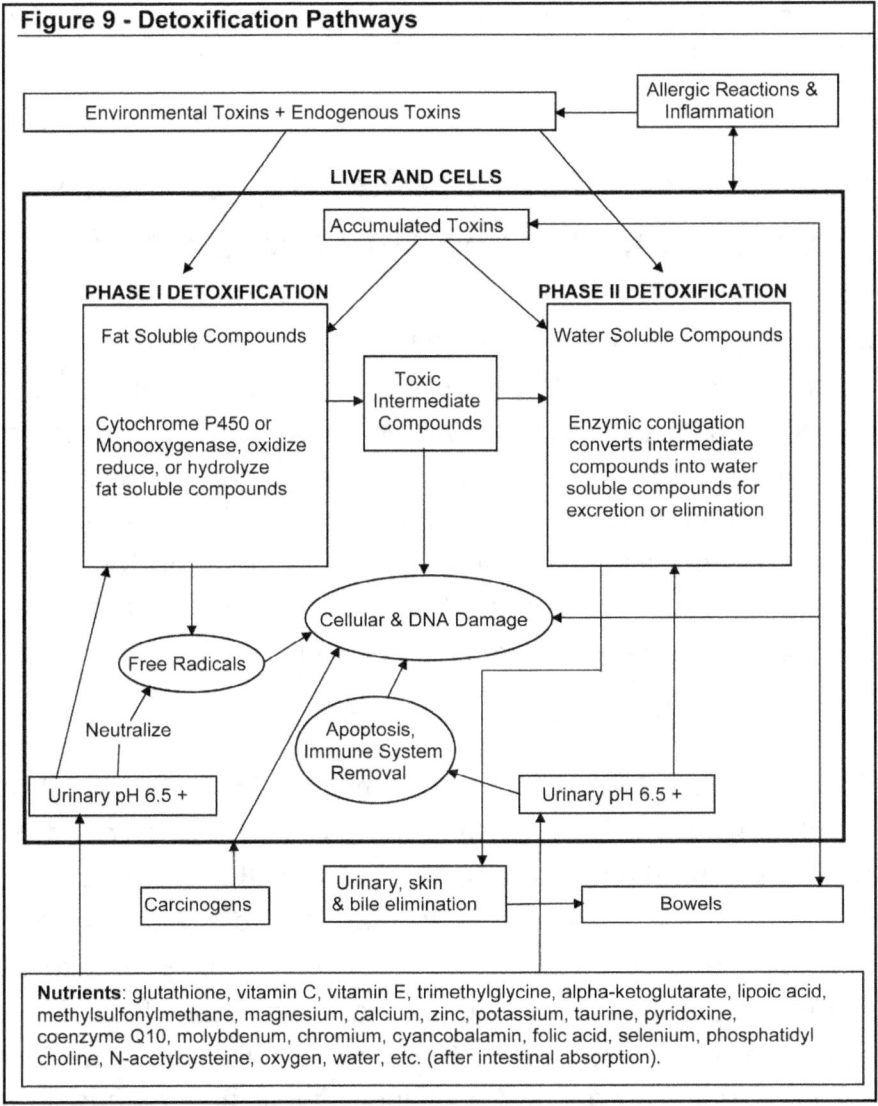

Figure 9 - Detoxification Pathways

Nutrients: glutathione, vitamin C, vitamin E, trimethylglycine, alpha-ketoglutarate, lipoic acid, methylsulfonylmethane, magnesium, calcium, zinc, potassium, taurine, pyridoxine, coenzyme Q10, molybdenum, chromium, cyancobalamin, folic acid, selenium, phosphatidyl choline, N-acetylcysteine, oxygen, water, etc. (after intestinal absorption).

Figure 9 – Detoxification Pathways demonstrates how the body accumulates toxins, which are fat-soluble and converts them into water soluble compounds that are excreted through the urine, bowel, and skin. The skin is a vitally important organ that eliminates toxins through

121

perspiration. Detoxification should be the first step in any comprehensive nutritional program.

Neurobiology Formula 12397 (NeuroLife) – Neurotransmitter and Glucose Control

5-Hydroxytryptophan should be taken in combination with other ingredients to raise levels of serotonin because there are other factors involved in raising serotonin and preventing the loss of serotonin. These factors need to be taken into consideration when developing a formula to raise the levels of serotonin and decrease the loss of serotonin. In migraines, depression, and other serotonin related disorders, norepinephrine plays an important role in a similar manor as does serotonin.

The patented Neurobiology Formula 12397 (NeuroLife), developed in 1997 by Dr. John A. Allocca, is designed to supply the nutrients required to facilitate the production of serotonin and norepinephrine in the brain, decrease allergic reactions, and control blood glucose levels. Daily intake of this formula will help to maintain the preventive effect of low serotonin disorders. Physicians have recommended this formula during pregnancy. The ingredients are: magnesium citrate, 5-Hydroxytryptophan, quercetin, calcium acorbate, zinc ctrate, inositol hexanicotinate, choline citrate, trimethylglycine HCl, alpha-lipoic acid, vanadyl sulfate, copper sebacate, chromium nicotinate, folic acid, vitamin D3.

The formula originally contained tyrosine. After clinical observations, the tyrosine was removed so that it could be titrated separately. After 10 years of clinical observations, the Neurobiology formula is undergoing a large scale trial in the "American Migraine Prevention Study."

5-Hydroxytryptophan is the precursor to serotonin. It should be taken with food to avoid nausea. Dosage greater than 300 mg can cause nausea with or without food.

Tyrosine is the precursor to norepinephrine and epinephrine, and thyroid hormones. copper and vitamin C are also required for the production of norepinephrine from tyrosine. Tyrosine can be synthesized in the body from phenylalanine, except in premature infants and in Phenylketonuria. Copper and vitamin C may be more important in supplementation than is tyrosine.

Magnesium is essential to the cellular metabolism of both carbohydrates and proteins because it is a significant cation (positive ion) of the intracellular fluid. It serves as an activator of many enzymes in the reactions of the initial glycogenic pathway of glucose oxidation. Magnesium is a coenzyme in protein synthesis. It is important in molecules formed in the process of growth and maintenance of tissues and is related to cortisone in the regulation of the blood phosphorus level. Decreased ionized magnesium concentration causes vasodilation and inhibits smooth muscle action. It is also essential for the maintenance of

DNA and RNA. Calcium and magnesium are required for normal nerve transmission. Magnesium and niacin are required for vasomotor control.

Calcium is the most abundant mineral in the body. To properly function, calcium must be accompanied by magnesium, phosphorus, vitamins A, C and D. Calcium is required for normal transmission of nerve impulses. Ionized calcium controls the passage of fluid through cell walls by affecting the cell wall permeability. Calcium ions are important activators of certain enzymes such as ATPase. In blood clotting, calcium ions enhance bonding between fibrin molecules and give stability to the fibrin threads. Ionized serum calcium plays an important role in the initiation of muscle contraction. Calcium is also necessary for acid-base equilibrium, heart regulation, and activation of metabolic hormones.

Niacin is used in the form of inositol hexanicotinate and niacinamide to minimize flushing and nausea associated with nicotinic acid. Niacin is used to insure that tryptophan is not converted to niacin instead of serotonin.

Quercetin is a bioflavonoid that strengthens outer cell membranes and help to stabilize the cell surface. It is used to stabilize the cell walls of basophils and mast cells, so they will not burst easily and release histamine and other inflammatory chemicals such as prostaglandins and leukotrienes. Prescription antihistamines can produce adverse side effects such as drowsiness, dry mouth, difficult urination, constipation, confusion, heart rhythm irregularities, nervousness, irritability, and more. Furthermore, antihistamines can inhibit the uptake of serotonin, norepinephrine and dopamine. For those who suffer from environmental allergies such as dust and pollen, quercetin is the treatment of choice, and it should be taken 3 times daily.

Vitamin C is a potent antioxidant. It is also required to convert pyridoxal dopamine to norepinephrine, l-tryptophan to 5-hydroxytryptophan, blocking delta-6-desaturase, and cyclooxygenase.

Pyridoxine (Vitamin B6) plays an important role in the production of neurotransmitters and prostaglandins. It is also important to inhibit tryptophan oxygenase, which metabolizes and depletes tryptophan.

Choline is a precursor for the neurotransmitter acetylcholine. It also increases the uptake of magnesium.

Trimethylglycine is a methyl donor. Methyl groups convert homocysteine, a toxic amino acid, to methionine, a beneficial amino acid. Methylation is required to convert norepinephrine to epinephrine. Methyl groups also attach to DNA and act in a protective capacity.

Alpha Lipoic Acid is a potent antioxidant that serves as a coenzyme in the citric acid cycle and in the production of cellular energy. Alpha-lipoic acid is converted into dihydrolipoic acid, which is a more powerful antioxidant than alpha-lipoic acid. Both forms of lipoic acid quench peroxynitrite radicals, an especially dangerous type consisting of both oxygen and nitrogen.

Folic acid (folacin) is a coenzyme of single carbon transfer. It is necessary for the synthesis of nucleic acids and certain amino acids, and the utilization of amino acids. It also participates in the reactions that synthesize thiamine, which is an essential nucleoprotein of DNA. Folic acid also facilitates the production of neurotransmitters.

Chromium is necessary for the utilization of sugars, involved with activity of hormones and enzymes, aids in metabolism of cholesterol, identified as a glucose tolerance factor, and helps to regulate serum cholesterol. Chromium regulates insulin action. It influences carbohydrate, lipid, and protein metabolism. Vanadium is essential for normal growth and makes insulin more efficient. Vanadium has an insulin-like effect in increasing glucose transport and metabolism. Chromium and vanadium help to stabilize glucose levels.

Zinc is a cofactor of the protein-splitting enzyme, carboxypeptidase. Zinc is also part of lactic dehydrogenase. Zinc combines readily with insulin in the pancreas. A significant quantity of zinc bound to protein is present in leukocytes. It is also essential for the synthesis of nucleic acids, normal prostrate function and helpful in healing wounds and burns. It is also vital for the synthesis of DNA and RNA. It aids the body in expelling carbon dioxide, normal growth, and tissue respiration. Unrefined cereal and breads contain phytates in the husks that inhibit the absorption of zinc. Zinc also plays a role in appetite control.

In 2002 the Eastern Virginia Medical School did an assessment / pilot study of patients who were treated with the Neurobiology 12397 formula for 1 year[50].

> "Effects of Neurobiology Formula on the Headaches of Chronic Migraineurs" Erin E. Icenbice, PA-S-Investigator, and Patricia Shull, PA-C, Co-Investigator Eastern Virginia Medical School, Norfolk, VA, June 2002.
>
> Abstract:
>
> Purpose: Neurobiology Formula 12397 is a relatively new and unexplored natural supplement intended for the prevention of migraine headaches. This research was done to see what effects, if any, the Formula has had on the lives of migraineurs who have taken it. Methods: A survey was mailed to 20 individuals across the United States who were known to take the Formula. Surveys contained questions addressing demographic information, migraine symptomatology, therapy course with Neurobiology formula, as well as effects on 6 dependent variables: days missed from work/

school, household work, and social events, severity of migraines, frequency of migraines, and impaired productivity. 15 surveys were returned complete. Results were analyzed using descriptive statistics. Results: Of the participating subjects, 93% were female and 60% older than 45 years of age. Most subjects (60%) were diagnosed with migraines before the age of 18. All participants claimed to experience at least one associated symptom during migraine attacks. Photophobia was reported by all participants, more than 70% of subjects reported suffering from phonophobia and nausea, and greater than 50% noted vomiting with their headaches. More than half of subjects had taken Neurobiology Formula for at least a year while the other half had taken the formula longer. No participants had taken the formula more than 3 years. Compliance with taking the formula was as follows: 26.7% never missed a dose, 46.7% rarely missed a dose, and 26.7% occasionally missed a dose. The dependent variables collectively showed positive results. Participants were asked to state the number of days in a three-month period that problems in question were encountered due to their migraines. Before taking Neurobiology Formula, over 30% of participants missed more than 10 days of work/school or social events. Over 40% missed household work more than 10 days. Impaired productivity on the job was encountered more than 10 days by over half of those surveyed. More than 70% stated they experienced greater than 10 headaches over this time period with an average severity of 8.7 on a scale of 1 to 10. Results concerning the time after subjects had started taking the formula were much different. Approximately 60% of those surveyed reported missing only 0-1 days of work/school, household work and social events over three months, while less than 10% reported missing more than 10 days. More than 40% of subjects experienced only 0-1 days of reduced productivity in the time surveyed. Additionally, subjects experienced fewer headaches with a majority (>50%) having less than 4 headaches over three months. Headache severity also reduced to an average of 4.3 on a scale of 1 to 10. Conclusions: There are limited prophylactic therapies for migraine sufferers. With approximately 28 million Americans coping with migraine pain and direct and indirect costs totaling near 17.2 million dollars annually for this condition, it is imperative to continue looking for helpful treatment regimens. This research was done to determine the effects of

Neurobiology Formula 12397 on chronic migraine headaches. It was hypothesized that those taking it would see positive changes in their headache pattern. Reviewing the analyzed results shows that this hypothesis was supported. With only 15 surveys to analyze, there is no way to state that this research is conclusive for the entire migraine population; however, the relief experienced by participants while taking the formula warrants further, more controlled research on this supplement.

Food to Avoid

Food Allergies

Eating any food you are allergic to can cause migraine headaches and other problems. If in doubt, see an allergist for food allergy testing. Food allergies may include, but not limited to the following:

Eggs, If allergic

Wheat, if allergic

Corn, if allergic

Milk, if allergic

Soy, if allergic

Anything else, if allergic

Tyramine Containing Food to Avoid

Food is fermented using bacteria, which produce tyramine, a chemical that causes migraine headaches and other problems. This includes the following.

Primary (absolutely avoid):

Any Food that is Aged, Cultured, Fermented, or naturally contains Tyramine

Cheeses

Chocolate

Yogurt

Over-ripened fruits

Citrus and Citric Acid

Secondary (small amounts may be tolerated):
Salt
Berries (most kinds with thick skin)
Red Plums
Pineapple
Raisins
Raspberries
Bananas
Grapes
Apples
Figs
Tomatoes
Raw Onions
Avocado
Spinach
Green Pepper
Chili Peppers
Nuts and nut butters
Coconut and coconut-oil
Many Beans and Peas
Frankfurters, bacon, etc. containing nitrates
Sourdough
Carob
Most teas are fermented
Garlic
Wine
Cold cuts containing nitrates, etc.
Salad bars that spray with sulfites
Aged, marinated, or pickled meats

Smoked/cured meats
Non-fresh meats or fish
Tofu
Smoked fish
Mustard
Red wine
Alcoholic beverages including beer
Caffeine greater than 300 mg per day
Tempeh
Tomari
Umbusi
Soy sauce
Miso
Vinegar
Tobacco
Protein extracts
Ginseng
Ginger

Chemicals to Avoid:

Monosodium Glutamate (MSG)

Nitrates & Nitrites

Meat tenderizers

Aspartame (nutrasweet)

Saccharin (includes toothpaste and mouthwash)

Food preservatives

Yeast and brewers extracts

Frequent use of amphetamines

Frequent use of barbituates

Frequent use of recreation drugs

Decaffeinated coffee (only 50% less caffeine)

Paint fumes & other chemical fumes

Some drugs can trigger a migraine, Depression, etc. depending upon ones sensitivity to those drugs

Excessive exposure to fluorescent lighting

Food to Eat

The following food are relatively safe to eat unless there is an allergy to any of them.

DIET IS NOT LIMITED TO THOSE ITEMS BELOW

Bell & Evans Frozen Fully Cooked Grilled Chicken Breasts, Frozen, Ingredients: boneless, skinless, chicken beasts, water, sea salt, rice starch.

Shiloh Farms Organic Potato Fakes, instant, Ingredients: organic potato flakes, monoglycerides, and diglycerides (from organic palm oil).

Any brand, Instant Oatmeal or regular oatmeal, Ingredients: whole grain instant oats.

Nature's Path Organic Crispy Rice, Ingredients: brown rice flour, evaporated cane juice, sea salt, molasses.

Nature's Path Organic Gorilla Munch Cereal, Ingredients: organic whole grain corn meal, organic corn meal, organic cane sugar, organic sea salt.

Quaker Rice Cakes, Ingredients: whole grain brown rice.

Romain Lettuce, broccoli, zucchini, carrots, and many other vegetables, except raw garlic, onions, and radishes.

Cold Pressed Olive Oil.

Coffee, unflavored, organic.

Organic Fat-Free Milk if not allergic.

Organic Butter in small quantities.

Ice Cream, vanilla.

Spices: parsley, oregano, basil, pepper, salt, in small quantity.

Sweetener: sugar in small quantity.

Brown Rice vs White Rice

Brown rice is the natural whole grain product with the outer husk (chaff) removed. White rice is raw rice product with the husk (chaff), bran, and cereal germ layers removed, leaving primarily the endosperm.

Many minerals and toxins are absorbed into the husk and bran layers of brown rice. The minerals and fiber in the bran are beneficial. The toxins that are absorbed by the bran can be harmful.

Arsenic is a toxic element naturally present in our environment. It is divided into two groups, organic and inorganic arsenic, with inorganic arsenic being more toxic. Rice accumulates more arsenic than other food crops. Long-term consumption may increase one's risk of chronic diseases including cancer, heart disease and type 2 diabetes. Brown rice tends to be higher in arsenic than white rice. A 2012 report from the US publication Consumer Reports found measurable levels of arsenic in nearly all of the 60 varieties of rice and rice products it tested in the US. Consumer Reports states that brown rice has 80 percent more inorganic arsenic on average than white rice of the same type, because the arsenic tends to accumulate in the outer layers of the grain. A 2013 analysis found that rice cereal and pasta can possess significantly more inorganic arsenic than the 2012 data showed; Consumer Reports said that just one serving of rice cereal or pasta could place children over the maximum amount of rice it recommended for their weekly allotment, due to arsenic content. One study published in the Proceedings of the National Academy of Sciences (US) journal found a median level of arsenic that was 56% higher in the urine of women who had eaten rice.

Toxins in rainwater and ground water are also absorbed into rice. What was once a nutritious product has become a depository of natural and man-made environmental toxins. Organic rice is certified to be free of pesticides and synthetic fertilizers. However, it is not free from toxins contained in rain water and ground water.

In summary, brown rice (organic or conventional) has a higher nutritional content and a higher toxin content. White rice (organic or conventional) has a lower nutritional content and a lower toxin content. Therefore, in this environment at this time, organic white rice would be the best choice.

Carbohydrate Balanced Meals

A meal should have more carbohydrate than fat. If daily meals consists of more fat than carbohydrate, the brain will not have a sufficient amount of glucose, resulting in the production of ketones from fat for the brain to survive. This is a process called "ketosis," which can lead to other problems. A high fat diet will require a high amount of carbohydrates. Therefore, a diabetic should seek a low fat, low carbohydrate diet. A carbohydrate content of 45%-60% is recommended.

The American Diabetes Foundation recommends 45-60 g carbohydrates per meal for adults.

A meal should contain more carbohydrate calories than fat calories.

1 gram fat = 9 calories
1 gram carbohydrate = 4 calories
1 gram protein = 4 calories

There is a carbohydrate balancing calculator in the library of www.allocca.com

Below are some balanced meal examples. An updated list can be found in the library of www.alloca.com

This chart provides the quantities of weight, fat, carbohydrate, protein, and calories for each meal. Each meal is designed to provide a adequate amount of balanced carbohydrate. A recommended scale is the American Weigh ONYX Slim Design Kitchen Scale. It is important to weigh the rice or potato for each meal.

The following are some examples of carbohydrate balanced meals.

Food	Weight (g)	Fat (g)	Carbohydrate (g)	Protein (g)	Calories
Items for Meals					
Apple, raw, no skin, (1 medium)	161.00	0.00	21.00	0.00	77.00
Butter, 1 pat (1" square x 1/3" high)	4.00	3.00	0.00	0.00	27.00
Cashew Flour 1 oz. (1/4 cup)	28.00	14.00	8.00	5.00	160.00
Cashew nuts, raw 1/4 cup (1 oz.)	28.00	14.00	8.00	5.00	160.00
Cashew nut butter (1 tablespoon)	15.00	7.50	4.50	2.00	90.00
Chicken breasts - grilled (1)	78.00	1.50	0.00	22.00	100.00
Chicken Curry	340.00	4.23	5.00	63.06	310.31
Coconut, raw (1 oz.)	28.00	9.00	4.00	1.00	99.00
Coconut, raw (1 tablespoon)	4.00	1.29	0.57	0.14	14.10
Corn flakes, lightly sweetened, 3/4 cup	30.00	0.00	27.00	2.00	110.00
Egg (1 large)	61.00	7.00	0.00	6.00	96.00
Granola, plain classic, Back to Nature brand, 1/2 cup	51.00	3.00	39.00	6.00	200.00
Granola, cranberry pecan, Back to Nature brand, 1/2 cup	47.00	4.50	36.00	3.00	180.00
Lentils, cooked, 1 cup	198.00	1.00	40.00	18.00	230.00
Oatmeal, Dry 1/2 cup	40.00	3.00	26.00	6.00	155.00
Oatmeal, cooked, 1 cup	234.00	4.00	32.00	6.00	188.00
Olive Oil (1 oz.)	28.00	28.00	0.00	0.00	252.00
Olive Oil (1 tablespoon)	14.00	14.00	0.00	0.00	126.00
Potato, baked	100.00	0.00	21.00	3.00	93.00
Potato, flakes, 1/3 cup	26.00	0.00	20.00	2.00	90.00
Potato, mashed with whole milk	210.00	1.00	37.00	4.00	210.00
Quinoa, cooked (1 cup)	185.00	4.00	39.00	8.00	224.00
Rice, white, california (1 cup)	186.00	0.00	53.00	4.00	242.00
Rice, cracker, white, sesame, 1	1.75	0.13	1.38	0.13	6.88

Food	Weight (g)	Fat (g)	Carbohydrate (g)	Protein (g)	Calories
Salad/Vegetables 2 cups	72.00	0.00	2.00	0.00	8.00
Sesame Seeds (1 cup)	144.00	72.00	34.00	26.00	825.00
Strawberry (1 medium)	12.00	0.00	1.00	0.00	4.00
Sugar, granular, 1 packet	3.50	0.00	4.00	0.00	15.00
Sunflower Oil (1 cup)	218.00	218.00	0.00	0.00	1,927.
Tomatoes, cooked (1 cup)	240.00	0.00	10.00	2.00	43.00
Tomato, raw (1 small)	91.00	0.00	4.00	1.00	16.00
Tomato Sauce, curry or Italian, with Olive Oil, 1 cup	247.00	7.00	10.00	2.00	106.00
Turkey (breast or dark meat)	170.00	2.80	7.20	29.00	176.00
Vegetable Curry	400.00	16.00	28.40	12.80	308.00
Brown rice has been removed from this meal plan because of recent findings (2012) of significant levels of arsenic in brown rice. White rice from california has much lower levels of arsenic.					

Food	Weight (g)	Fat (g)	Carbohydrate (g)	Protein (g)	Calories
A meal should have more carbohydrate than fat. If daily meals consists of more fat than carbohydrate, the brain will not have a sufficient amount of glucose, resulting in the production of ketones from fat for the brain to survive. This is a process called "ketosis," which can lead to other problems. A high fat diet will require a high amount of carbohydrates. Therefore, a diabetic should seek a low fat, low carbohydrate diet. A carbohydrate content of 45%-60% is recommended.					
The Gluten Test The first step is to measure blood glucose levels 2 hours after meals while avoiding all gluten products for 4 days. Re-introduce a gluten product, such as wheat, containing the same amount of carbohydrates, during a specific meal. Measure the blood glucose level after 2 hours. Compare the readings with and without gluten. Repeat this process several times. Blood glucose meters can be purchased at local pharmacies.					

Food	Weight (g)	Fat (g)	Carbohydrate (g)	Protein (g)	Calories
The Dairy Test The first step is to measure blood glucose levels 2 hours after meals while avoiding all dairy products for 4 days. Re-introduce a dairy product, such as milk during a specific meal. Measure the blood glucose level after 2 hours. Compare the readings with and without dairy. Repeat this process several times. Blood glucose meters can be purchased at local pharmacies.					
American Diabetes Foundation recommends 45-60 grams carbohydrates per meal for adults					
A meal should contain more carbohydrate calories than fat calories.					
1 gram fat = 9 calories					
1 gram carbohydrate = 4 calories					
1 gram protein = 4 calories					

Food	Weight (g)	Fat (g)	Carbohydrate (g)	Protein (g)	Calories
This chart provides the quantities of weight, fat, carbohydrate, protein, and calories for each meal. Each meal is designed to provide a adequate amount of balanced carbohydrate. A recommended scale is the American Weigh ONYX Slim Design Kitchen Scale. It is important to weigh the rice or potato for each meal.					
Snack					
Cashew nuts, raw 1/2 cup (1 oz.)	56.00	28.00	16.00	10.00	320.00
Totals: Fat-70.79%, Carb-17.98%, Protein-11.24%	56.00	28.00	16.00	10.00	320.00
Snack					
Apple, raw, no skin, (1 medium)	161.00	0.00	21.00	0.00	77.00
Totals: Carb-100%	161.00	0.00	21.00	0.00	77.00
Snack					
Apple, raw, no skin, (1 medium)	161.00	0.00	21.00	0.00	77.00
Cashew Flour or Cashew nuts	23.80	11.90	6.80	4.25	151.30
Cold water	0.00	0.00	0.00	0.00	0.00
Totals: Fat-45.52%, Carb-47.26%, Protein-7.22%	184.80	11.90	27.80	4.25	235.30

Food	Weight (g)	Fat (g)	Carbohydrate (g)	Protein (g)	Calories
Snack - Apple Cashew Dessert					
5 medium Apples, raw, no skin	805.00	0.00	105.00	0.00	385.00
1/2 cup Cashew nuts	69.51	34.76	19.86	12.42	441.90
1/2 cup Cashew flour	53.51	26.76	15.29	9.56	340.18
4 tablespoons unsweetened shredded coconut	16.00	5.16	2.28	0.56	56.40
4 Strawberries	48.00	0.00	4.00	0.00	16.00
1-1/4 cups water	0.00	0.00	0.00	0.00	0.00
Totals: Fat-47.04%, Carb-45.90%, Protein-7.07%	992.02	66.68	146.43	22.54	1,239.
Divide recipe by 4			36.61		
Snack					
Granola, plain classic, Back to Nature brand	23.59	1.39	18.04	2.78	95.79
Cold water	0.00	0.00	0.00	0.00	0.00
Totals: Fat-13.06%, Carb-75.35%, Protein-11.59%	23.59	1.39	18.04	2.78	95.79
Snack					
Granola, plain classic, Back to Nature brand	39.23	2.31	30.00	4.62	159.27
Cold water	0.00	0.00	0.00	0.00	0.00
Totals: Fat-13.06%, Carb-75.35%, Protein-11.59%	39.23	2.31	30.00	4.62	159.27

Food	Weight (g)	Fat (g)	Carbohydrate (g)	Protein (g)	Calories
Snack					
Granola, plain classic, Back to Nature brand	47.18	2.78	36.08	5.55	191.54
Cold water	0.00	0.00	0.00	0.00	0.00
Totals: Fat-13.06%, Carb-75.35%, Protein-11.59%	47.18	2.78	36.08	5.55	191.54
Snack					
Rice, cracker, white, sesame, 1	1.75	0.13	1.38	0.13	6.88
Cashew nut butter (1/4 teaspoon)	1.25	3.75	0.38	0.17	7.50
Totals: Fat-%, Carb-%, Protein-%	3.00	3.88	1.75	0.30	14.38
10 crackers with cashew nut butter	30.00	38.80	17.50	3.00	143.80
Snack					
Corn flakes, lightly sweetened	20.01	0.00	18.01	1.33	77.36
Cold water	0.00	0.00	0.00	0.00	0.00
Totals: Fat-0%, Carb-93.12%, Protein-6.88%	20.01	0.00	18.01	1.33	77.36
Snack					
Corn flakes, lightly sweetened	33.36	0.00	30.02	2.22	128.96
Cold water	0.00	0.00	0.00	0.00	0.00
Totals: Fat-0%, Carb-93.12%, Protein-6.88%	33.36	0.00	30.02	2.22	128.96
Snack					

Food	Weight (g)	Fat (g)	Carbohydrate (g)	Protein (g)	Calories
Corn flakes, lightly sweetened	40.05	0.00	36.05	2.67	154.88
Cold water	0.00	0.00	0.00	0.00	0.00
Totals: Fat-0%, Carb-93.12%, Protein-6.88%	40.05	0.00	36.05	2.67	154.88
Breakfast					
Oatmeal, Dry	69.24	5.19	45.01	10.39	268.31
Hot water	0.00	0.00	0.00	0.00	0.00
Totals: Fat-17.41%, Carb-67.10%, Protein-15.49%	69.24	5.19	45.01	10.39	268.31
Breakfast					
Oatmeal, Dry	63.20	3.16	41.08	9.48	230.68
Sugar, granular, 1 packet	3.50	0.00	4.00	0.00	15.00
Hot water	0.00	0.00	0.00	0.00	0.00
Totals: Fat-11.53%, Carb-73.10%, Protein-15.37%	66.70	3.16	45.08	9.48	246.68
Breakfast					
Oatmeal, cooked	329.24	5.63	45.02	8.44	264.51
Totals: Fat-19.16%, Carb-68.08%, Protein-12.76%	329.24	5.63	45.02	8.44	264.51
Breakfast					

Food	Weight (g)	Fat (g)	Carbohydrate (g)	Protein (g)	Calories
Oatmeal, cooked	300.23	5.13	41.06	7.70	241.21
Sugar, granular, 1 packet	3.50	0.00	4.00	0.00	15.00
Totals: Fat-17.95%, Carb-70.08%, Protein-11.97%	303.73	5.13	45.06	7.70	257.21
Breakfast					
Granola, plain classic, Back to Nature brand	58.91	3.47	45.05	6.93	239.15
Cold water	0.00	0.00	0.00	0.00	0.00
Totals: Fat-13.06%, Carb-75.35%, Protein-11.59%	58.91	3.47	45.05	6.93	239.15
Breakfast					
Granola, plain classic, Back to Nature brand	48.45	2.85	37.05	5.70	196.65
Cashew Flour or Cashew nuts	28.00	14.00	8.00	5.00	178.00
Cold water	0.00	0.00	0.00	0.00	0.00
Totals: Fat-40.08%, Carb-48.10%, Protein-11.42%	76.45	16.85	45.05	10.70	374.65
Breakfast					
Corn flakes, lightly sweetened	40.05	0.00	36.05	2.67	154.88
Cashew Flour or Cashew nuts	31.64	15.82	9.04	5.65	201.14
Cold water	0.00	0.00	0.00	0.00	0.00
Totals: Fat-39.99%, Carb-50.66%, Protein-9.35%	71.69	15.82	45.09	8.32	356.02
Lunch					

Food	Weight (g)	Fat (g)	Carbohydrate (g)	Protein (g)	Calories
Chicken breasts - grilled (2) with white Rice	156.00	3.00	0.00	44.00	203.00
Rice, white, california	155.31	0.00	45.04	3.11	192.60
Olive Oil (1 tablespoon)	14.00	14.00	0.00	0.00	126.00
Totals: Fat-29.33%, Carb-34.54%, Protein-36.13%	325.30	17.00	45.04	47.11	421.60
Lunch					
Chicken breasts - grilled (2) with Potato	156.00	3.00	0.00	44.00	203.00
Potato, baked	214.50	0.00	45.05	6.44	205.96
Olive Oil (1 tablespoon)	14.00	14.00	0.00	0.00	126.00
Totals: Fat-28.6%, Carb-33.68%, Protein-37.71%	384.50	17.00	45.05	50.44	534.96
Lunch					
Chicken breasts - grilled (2) with Potato	156.00	3.00	0.00	44.00	203.00
Potato, flakes	58.50	0.00	45.00	4.50	198.00
Hot water	0.00	0.00	0.00	0.00	0.00
Olive Oil (1 tablespoon)	14.00	14.00	0.00	0.00	126.00
Totals: Fat-29.03%, Carb-34.16%, Protein-36.81%	228.50	17.00	45.00	48.50	527.00
Lunch					
Lentils, cooked	225.75	1.13	45.00	20.25	271.17
Totals: Fat-3.75%, Carb-66.38%, Protein-29.87%	225.75	1.13	45.00	20.25	271.17

Food	Weight (g)	Fat (g)	Carbohydrate (g)	Protein (g)	Calories
Dinner					
Chicken breasts - grilled (2) with white Rice & Salad	156.00	3.00	0.00	44.00	200.00
Rice, white, california	148.43	0.00	43.04	2.97	184.04
Salad/Vegetables 2 cups	72.00	0.00	2.00	0.00	8.00
Olive Oil (1 tablespoon)	14.00	14.00	0.00	0.00	126.00
Totals: Fat-29.36%, Carb-34.58%, Protein-36.06%	390.40	17.00	45.04	46.97	521.04
Dinner					
Chicken breasts - grilled (2) with Potato & Salad	156.00	3.00	0.00	44.00	200.00
Potato, baked	204.80	0.00	43.01	6.14	196.60
Salad/Vegetables 2 cups	72.00	0.00	2.00	0.00	8.00
Olive Oil (1 tablespoon)	14.00	14.00	0.00	0.00	126.00
Totals: Fat-28.67%, Carb-33.74%, Protein-37.59%	446.80	17.00	45.01	50.14	533.60
Dinner					
Chicken breasts - grilled (2) with Potato & Salad	156.00	3.00	0.00	44.00	200.00
Potato, flakes	55.90	0.00	43.00	4.30	189.20
Hot water	0.00	0.00	0.00	0.00	0.00
Salad/Vegetables 2 cups	72.00	0.00	2.00	0.00	8.00
Olive Oil (1 tablespoon)	14.00	14.00	0.00	0.00	126.00
Totals: Fat-29.08%, Carb-34.21%, Protein-36.72%	297.90	17.00	45.00	48.30	526.20

Food	Weight (g)	Fat (g)	Carbohydrate (g)	Protein (g)	Calories
Dinner					
Chicken Curry (Indian Restaurant)	340.00	4.23	5.00	63.06	310.31
Rice, white	138.01	0.00	40.02	2.23	169.00
Totals: Fat-7.94%, Carb-37.57%, Protein-54.49%	478.01	4.23	45.02	65.29	479.31
Dinner					
Vegetable Curry (Indian Restaurant)	320.00	12.80	22.72	10.24	247.04
Rice, white	77.00	0.00	22.33	1.54	95.48
Totals: Fat-14.11%, Carb-80.71%, Protein-5.18%	397.00	12.80	45.05	11.78	342.52
Dinner					
Chicken breast - grilled - Sweet Mama's Restaurant	174.00	3.35	0.00	49.06	226.39
Vegetables	345.60	0.00	9.60	0.00	48.00
Potato, baked	169.00	0.00	35.49	5.07	162.24
Totals: Fat-7.06%, Carb-42.24%, Protein-50.70%	688.60	3.35	45.09	54.13	427.03
Dinner					
Chicken breasts - grilled - Pumpernickel's Restaurant	160.00	3.08	0.00	45.14	208.28
Salad/Vegetables 2 cups	72.00	0.00	2.00	0.00	8.00
Mashed Potatoes with milk	244.44	1.16	43.07	4.66	201.36
Totals: Fat-9.14%, Carb-43.17%, Protein-47.70%	467.50	4.24	45.07	49.80	417.64

Food	Weight (g)	Fat (g)	Carbohydrate (g)	Protein (g)	Calories
Dinner					
Turkey (breast or dark meat) with Brown Rice	170.00	2.80	7.20	29.00	170.00
Salad/Vegetables 2 cups	72.00	0.00	2.00	0.00	8.00
Rice, white, california	123.50	0.00	35.82	2.47	153.16
Olive Oil (1 tablespoon)	14.00	14.00	0.00	0.00	126.00
Totals: Fat-33.07%, Carb-39.39%, Protein-27.54%	379.50	16.80	45.02	31.47	457.16
Dinner					
Turkey (breast or dark meat) with Potato	170.00	2.80	7.20	29.00	170.00
Salad/Vegetables 2 cups	72.00	0.00	2.00	0.00	8.00
Potato, baked	170.50	0.00	35.81	5.12	163.72
Olive Oil (1 tablespoon)	14.00	14.00	0.00	0.00	126.00
Totals: Fat-32.33%, Carb-38.49%, Protein-29.18%	426.50	16.80	45.01	34.12	467.72
Dinner					
Turkey drumstick (456g total, 267 g meat) with Potato	267.00	4.40	11.30	45.53	266.92
Salad/Vegetables 2 cups	72.00	0.00	2.00	0.00	8.00
Potato, baked	151.00	0.00	31.71	4.53	144.96
Olive Oil (1 tablespoon)	14.00	14.00	0.00	0.00	126.00
Totals: Fat-30.34%, Carb-32.98%, Protein-36.68%	504.00	18.40	45.01	50.06	545.88

Food	Weight (g)	Fat (g)	Carbohydrate (g)	Protein (g)	Calories
This document is available in the library of www.allocca.com	1/12/1				
There is a Carbohydrate Balancing Calculator in the library of www.allocca.com					

Gluten and Dairy

Gluten (wheat, kamut, spelt, barley, rye, and triticale) and dairy may not be suitable for individuals with celiac disease and autoimmune disorders such as type 1 diabetes. Gluten and dairy in individuals with autoimmune disorder can inhibit the absorption of cysteine. Cysteine is an amino acid that is the precursor to glutathione, a powerful antioxidant. There are also immune reactions to gluten and dairy among many people. It is wise to try a gluten and dairy free diet.

The Gluten Sensitivity Test

The first step is to measure blood glucose levels 2 hours after meals while avoiding all gluten products for 4 days. Re-introduce a gluten product, such as wheat, containing the same amount of carbohydrates, during a specific meal. Measure the blood glucose level after 2 hours. Compare the readings with and without gluten. Repeat this process several times. Blood glucose meters can be purchased at local pharmacies.

The Dairy Sensitivity Test

The first step is to measure blood glucose levels 2 hours after meals while avoiding all dairy products for 4 days. Re-introduce a dairy product, such as milk during a specific meal. Measure the blood glucose level after 2 hours. Compare the readings with and without dairy. Repeat this process several times. Blood glucose meters can be purchased at local pharmacies.

A significant rise in blood glucose after ingestion of a substance compared to normal blood glucose levels indicates a sensitivity to the substance tested.

Caffeine

Caffeine has a detrimental effect on the body, especially the cardiovascular system. Caffeine may also mask ones true energy level. Many people do not have enough energy to function without a substantial amount coffee every day. Caffeine is also addictive. The more caffeine one drinks, the more caffeine ones body will require for the same effect. If you are eating properly, and are in good health, you will not require the stimulation of caffeine to feel energetic.

A 5-ounce cup of coffee contains approximately 190 mg caffeine. A cup of tea varies from 10 to 90 mg. Regular use of more than 350 mg of caffeine per day causes physical dependence. 1 cup of coffee per day is not likely to cause addiction. Limit the intake of caffeine to not more than 250 mg per day.

If the intake of caffeine is more than 250 mg per day, A slow withdrawal will be required from the caffeine addiction. For example, if you are consuming 6 cups of coffee per day, cut this down to 5 cups per day for 4 days, then 4 cups per day for 4 days, then 3 cups per day for 4 days, then 2 cups per day for 4 days, then 1 cup per day for 4 days. Do not exercise during this withdrawal period.

Caffeine Content of Foods and Drugs

Product	Serving Size	Caffeine (mg)

OTC Drugs

Product	Serving Size	Caffeine (mg)
NoDoz, maximum strength; Vivarin	1 tablet	200
Excedrin	2 tablets	130
NoDoz, regular strength	1 tablet	100
Anacin	2 tablets	64

Coffee

Product	Serving Size	Caffeine (mg)
Coffee, brewed	8 oz.	135
General Foods International Coffee, Orange Cappuccino	8 oz.	102
Coffee, instant	8 oz.	95
General Foods International Coffee, Cafe Vienna	8 oz.	90
Maxwell House Cappuccino, Mocha	8 oz.	60-65
General Foods International Coffee, Swiss Mocha	8 oz.	55
Maxwell House Cappuccino, French Vanilla or Irish Cream	8 oz.	45-50
House Cappuccino, Amaretto	8 oz.	25-30
General Foods International Coffee, Viennese Chocolate Café	8 oz.	26
Maxwell House Cappuccino, decaffeinated	8 oz.	3-6
Coffee, decaffeinated	8 oz.	5

Product	Serving Size	Caffeine (mg)

Tea

Product	Serving Size	Caffeine (mg)
Bigelow Raspberry Royale Tea	8 oz.	83
Tea, leaf or bag	8 oz.	50
Snapple Iced Tea, all varieties	16-oz.	42
Lipton Natural Brew Iced Tea Mix, unsweetened	8 oz.	25-45
Lipton Tea	8 oz.	35-40
Lipton Iced Tea, assorted varieties	16-oz.	18-40
Lipton Natural Brew Iced Tea Mix, sweetened	8 oz.	15-35
Nestea Pure Sweetened Iced Tea	16-oz.	34
Tea, green	8 oz.	30
Arizona Iced Tea, assorted varieties	16-oz.	15-30
Lipton Soothing Moments Blackberry Tea	8 oz.	25
Tea, instant	8 oz.	15
Lipton Natural Brew Iced Tea Mix, diet	8 oz.	10-15
Lipton Natural Brew Iced Tea Mix, Decaffeinated	8 oz.	< 5
Celestial Seasonings Herbal Tea, all varieties	8 oz.	0
Celestial Seasonings Herbal Iced Tea, bottled	16-oz.	0
Lipton Soothing Moments Peppermint Tea	8 oz.	0

Product	Serving Size	Caffeine (mg)

Soft Drinks

Product	Serving Size	Caffeine (mg)
Josta	12 oz.	58
Mountain Dew	12 oz.	55.5
Surge	12 oz.	52.5
Diet Coke	12 oz.	46.5
Coca-Cola Classic	12 oz.	34.5
Dr. Pepper, regular or diet	12 oz.	42
Sunkist Orange Soda	12 oz.	42
Pepsi-Cola	12 oz.	37.5
Barqs Root Beer	12 oz.	22.5
7-UP or Diet 7-UP	12 oz.	0
Barqs Diet Root Beer	12 oz.	0
Caffeine-free Coca-Cola or Diet Coke	12 oz.	0
Caffeine-free Pepsi or Diet Pepsi	12 oz.	0
Minute Maid Orange Soda	12 oz.	0
Mug Root Beer	12 oz.	0
Sprite or Diet Sprite	12 oz.	0

Caffeinated Waters

Product	Serving Size	Caffeine (mg)
Java Water (1/2 liter)	16.9 oz.	125
Krank 20 (1/2 liter)	16.9 oz.	100
Aqua Blast (1/2 liter)	16.9 oz.	90
Water Joe (1/2 liter)	16.9 oz.	60-70
Aqua Java (1/2 liter)	16.9 oz.	50-60

Product	Serving Size	Caffeine (mg)

Frozen Desserts

Product	Serving Size	Caffeine (mg)
Ben & Jerry's No Fat Coffee Fudge Frozen Yogurt	1 cup	85
Starbucks Coffee Ice Cream, assorted flavors	1 cup	40-60
Häagen-Dazs Coffee Ice Cream	1 cup	58
Häagen-Dazs Coffee Frozen Yogurt, fat-free	1 cup	40
Häagen-Dazs Coffee Fudge Ice Cream, low-fat	1 cup	30
Starbucks Frappuccino Bar	1 bar (2.5 oz.)	15
Healthy Choice Cappuccino Chocolate Chunk or Cappuccino Mocha Fudge Ice Cream	1 cup	8
Yogurt, one container:		
Dannon Coffee Yogurt	8 oz.	45
Yoplait Cafe Au Lait Yogurt	6 oz.	5
Dannon Light Cappuccino Yogurt	8 oz.	< 1
Stonyfield Farm Cappuccino Yogurt	8 oz.	0

Chocolates or Candies

Product	Serving Size	Caffeine (mg)
Hershey's Special Dark Chocolate Bar	1 bar (1.5 oz.)	31
Perugina Milk Chocolate Cappuccino Filling	1/3 bar (1.2 oz.)	24
Hershey Bar (milk chocolate)	1 bar (1.5 oz.)	10
Coffee Nips (hard candy)	2 pieces	6
Cocoa or Hot Chocolate	8 oz.	5

Tea

Drinking tea began 5,000 years ago in China. It soon spread to Japan. Tea drinking reached Europe in the mid-16th century, when Dutch merchants discovered tea in their search for precious spices. Tea soon became the most popular beverage in Britain and much of Europe. Today, tea is the most popular beverage in the world next to water. In addition to the soothing, meditative qualities of tea, there is increasing evidence for the health benefits of tea drinking. Recent studies show tea may lower blood pressure and cholesterol, stabilize blood sugar and destroy decay-causing bacteria. The antioxidants in tea give it the potential to inhibit the development of cardiovascular diseases and certain cancers.

There are three basic types of tea: black, green, and oolong. Green tea is the least processed, whereby the leaves are steamed, rolled and dried. Black tea undergoes the most processing, whereby the leaves are allowed to ferment, beginning with a withering process. Then they are rolled, left to oxidize then, dried. Oolong tea is semi-fermented, which makes it stronger than green tea but weaker than black tea. Herbal teas and fruit teas are not actually teas as they do not contain tea leaves, and therefore no caffeine. Tea absorbs moisture and odors easily. It should be kept in its original container or air tight containers. Drinking tea that is high in caffeine is not recommended.

Approximate caffeine contents per 5 ounce cup are:

Coffee - 190 mg
Oolong tea - 50 mg
Black tea - 105 mg
Green tea - 30 mg
Herbal tea - none

Summary

When examining levels of neurotransmitters, it must be done with respect to time. Changes in neurotransmitter levels begin with an initial reaction followed by a loss of neurotransmitter reserves if they cannot be replaced at least at the same rate by which they are depleted.

Serotonin is somewhat difficult for the body to manufacture as the raw materials are not always found readily in the diet. Additionally, there are a number of environmental and dietary factors that cause the loss of serotonin. Serotonin and norepinephrine related disorders affect not only the individual who suffers from it, but the family, friends, and members of the community.

Norepinephrine is tricky to balance. A low level can cause depression and migraine headaches. A higher than normal amount can cause insomnia. A very high level can cause increased aggression, anger, and often violence.

There is a significant number of low serotonin and norepinephrine related disorders:
- Migraine headaches
- Depression
- Insomnia
- Bipolar syndrome
- Increased anger and outbursts
- Increased aggression
- Anxiety disorder
- Moodiness and socially withdrawal
- Increased escape fantasies and need for change
- Decreased sexuality
- Increased body temperature
- Increased appetite for carbohydrates
- Irritable bowel syndrome
- Tinnitus
- Fibromyalgia
- Premenstrual syndrome (PMS)
- Seasonal affective disorder (SAD).

There are a number of causes of serotonin and norepinephrine imbalance:
- Not enough tryptophan or 5-Hydroxytryptophan related chemicals to produce serotonin and norepinephrine
- Chemical depletion
- Tyramine depletion
- Inflammatory eicosanoids
- Allergic reactions
- Emotional Stress and Alcohol

- Changes in gonadatropin hormone levels
- Increased psychological anxiety
- Intestinal dysbiosis
- Dehydration
- High glycemic diet

Serotonin and norepinephrine levels can be balanced by, avoiding the foods on the "Avoid Foods" list, eating low glycemic index foods, drinking plenty of water, supplementation to provide the brain with the nutrients it needs to make serotonin and norepinephrine, decrease allergic reactions, and control glucose levels, supplementation to control gonadatropin hormone levels in men and women over 40, bowel cleansing and detoxification, liver detoxification, destroying harmful microorganisms in the intestinal tract, replenishing lactobacillus bifidus and lactobacillus acidophilus intestinal flora, additional nutrients to decrease seasonal allergic reactions, additional Nutrients to decrease inflammatory eicosanoids, melatonin to decrease serotonin load, general health supplementation, stress reduction, and following the multi-week step by step protocol.

Unfortunately, life, ailments, and treatments are not simple. This book illustrates the extreme complexity of serotonin and norepinephrine loss and treatment required to raise those levels. Consequently, the treatment protocol needs to comprise of a comprehensive nutritional program that includes a food dietary program, supplements, and a lifestyle change, if possible.

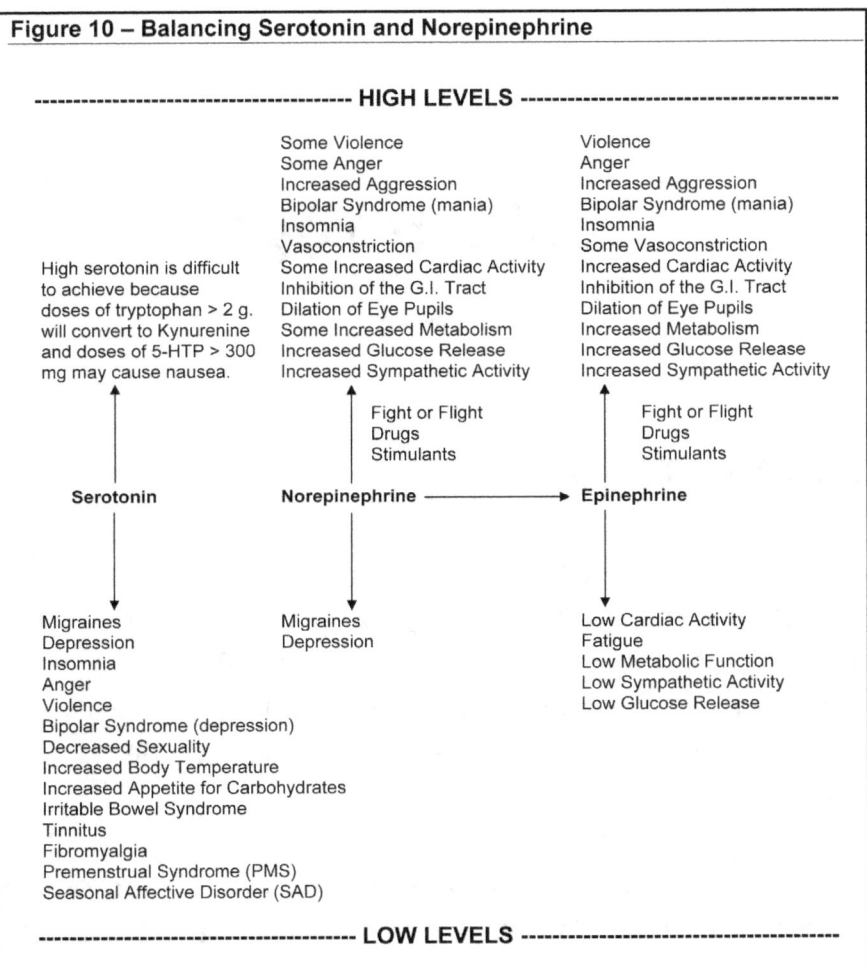

Figure 10 – Balancing Serotonin and Norepinephrine

-- HIGH LEVELS --

High serotonin is difficult
to achieve because
doses of tryptophan > 2 g.
will convert to Kynurenine
and doses of 5-HTP > 300
mg may cause nausea.

Some Violence
Some Anger
Increased Aggression
Bipolar Syndrome (mania)
Insomnia
Vasoconstriction
Some Increased Cardiac Activity
Inhibition of the G.I. Tract
Dilation of Eye Pupils
Some Increased Metabolism
Increased Glucose Release
Increased Sympathetic Activity

Violence
Anger
Increased Aggression
Bipolar Syndrome (mania)
Insomnia
Some Vasoconstriction
Increased Cardiac Activity
Inhibition of the G.I. Tract
Dilation of Eye Pupils
Increased Metabolism
Increased Glucose Release
Increased Sympathetic Activity

Fight or Flight
Drugs
Stimulants

Fight or Flight
Drugs
Stimulants

Serotonin   **Norepinephrine** ⟶ **Epinephrine**

Migraines
Depression
Insomnia
Anger
Violence
Bipolar Syndrome (depression)
Decreased Sexuality
Increased Body Temperature
Increased Appetite for Carbohydrates
Irritable Bowel Syndrome
Tinnitus
Fibromyalgia
Premenstrual Syndrome (PMS)
Seasonal Affective Disorder (SAD)

Migraines
Depression

Low Cardiac Activity
Fatigue
Low Metabolic Function
Low Sympathetic Activity
Low Glucose Release

-- LOW LEVELS --

Notes: The effects of epinephrine last 5-10 times longer and have a greater effect on metabolism and cardiac stimulation than norepinephrine, and have a weaker effect on vasoconstriction / increased blood pressure. The dynamics of neurotransmitter levels must be analyzed with respect to time. Changes in neurotransmitter levels begins with an initial reaction followed by a loss of neurotransmitter reserves if they cannot be replaced at least at the rate by which they are depleted.

Figure 10 – Balancing Serotonin and Norepinephrine, shows the various pathologies associated with low serotonin and norepinephrine. It is not just a matter of raising both as this could lead to undesirable effects such as increased aggression and violence. Serotonin can be high, if a high level can be achieved, which is difficult, without creating adverse effects. However norepinephrine should not be high or low because these levels can cause pathologies.

Desktop Yoga

What is Yoga?

According to the teachings of yoga, human nature is divine, perfect, and infinite. However, people are not aware of this because they falsely identify themselves with objects of the external world. This false identification makes people believe they are imperfect, limited, subject to sorrow, decay, and death.

The techniques of yoga provide us with the tools to enable us to cast off this false belief and become aware of our own true self, which is pure and free from imperfections. The process of yoga is to unite the individual self with the Universal Self. It is a journey of ascension into the purity of absolute perfection, which is the original state of human-kind. To accomplish this, one must remove the impurities in both body and mind so that the true Self can shine through. Yoga is the process of removing thoughts from the mind so that it can focus on a single point and turn inward towards the center of consciousness. The mind cannot be totally separated from the body because one influences the other. A sound mind can only thrive in a health body. Conversely, a body cannot thrive without a healthy mind. The ancient yogis developed the techniques of asana and pranayama (postures and breathing) in combination with meditation to cleanse the body and strengthen the nervous system.

Yoga is a powerful tool for releasing the fear and anger locked in the body's tissues, reducing cravings, and addictions.

When one's heart is open and you are experiencing turmoil around you, it can be devastating. Meditation practice gives us the tools for letting it in without getting swept away by it. In yoga, the journey "is" the destination.

What is Desktop Yoga?

Desktop Yoga is a modern style for those who have little time and for those who have little energy

One of the primary purposes of yoga and meditation is to "still" the mind. This was difficult even for the sages that developed yoga. Today's society is 100 times more stressful than our grandparents. With radio, television, computers, e-mail, cell phones, and other technologies, minds are constantly being stressed. When traditional yoga is performed in a stressful society, the stressful mind may continue to "chatter," even within the postures. Furthermore, most people don't have the time to practice yoga.

The Desktop Yoga style was developed by Dr. John A. Allocca in response to the growing need for a yoga style that can be performed successfully in a stressful society. It brings the scattered, stressful, chattering, mind into focus by integrating coordinated breathing and slow movements within each posture. The mind must focus its attention on coordinating the breathing and slow movements, which removes it's attention from the "chatter." The result is a yoga practice that "stills" the mind and creates relaxation. The bilateral movements are also designed to stimulate the release of stored emotional traumas from the limbic system in the brain, creating a greater sense of peace and well-being. The slow movements thin the fluid in the joints and allow even better stretching than postures without movements. Desktop yoga can be performed while sitting in an armless chair. It is a low-intensity, short-duration series of postures for those who have little time and for those who have little energy. The routine will take approximately 15 minutes to perform, not including the meditation.

Breathing

Sit straight facing forward with your feet together.

Slowly and deeply inhale from your abdomen first, then your chest.

Slowly exhale completely and push from your abdomen.

During Asanas, you can keep your eyes closed or open. I prefer closed. I prefer to take 3 slow, deep breaths for each posture. Three breaths will take about 15 seconds. As you advance, your breaths can be longer.

Relaxing Into A Posture

Don't push your muscles into a stretch. Allow them to stretch by relaxing your muscles. Don't stretch to the point of pain. If you experience pain, release a little or come out of the posture.

Counting Your Breaths

I count my breaths by saying (mentally) "Om" during the inhalation and the number during the exhalation. For example, Om (inhale), one (exhale), Om (inhale), two (exhale), Om (inhale), three (exhale). If you are in a group, just say (mentally) Om (inhale), then (exhale) and allow the instructor to tell you when to release.

Movement Cycles

All movements should be done slowly while concentrating on your breaths. Do not move quickly. This is not an aerobic exercise. If, for example, you are rotating your head from center to the left, you should inhale as you are rotating your head. The inhalation should take the entire time that you are slowly rotating.

Warm-up Exercises

Rubbing Hands

Rub hands together vigorously.

Neck Roll

Roll neck clockwise one complete rotation. Roll neck counter clockwise one complete rotation. Repeat 3 times.

Small Arm Circles

Hands and arms out to the side. Make small circular rotations with hands 3 times. Reverse direction and repeat 3 times.

Shoulder Roll

Roll shoulders forward 3 times.
Roll shoulders backward 3 times.
Lift shoulders up and down 3 times.

Waist Twisting

Arms horizontal and to the front at shoulder level. Rotate from side to side, keeping head and hips forward 3 times.

Arms Up and Down

Inhale, arms to the front and up to the sky. Exhale arms down to the side. Repeat 3 times.

Horizontal Adduction Arm Cross

Arms out to the sides. Then move to the front and back, alternating which hand is on top each time. Repeat 3 times.

Desktop Yoga Postures (Asanas)

Neck Rotation Posture

Sit straight facing forward with your feet together.

Inhale deeply.

- a. Exhale as you slowly rotate your head to the left while pushing your chin gently with your right hand.

- b. Inhale as you slowly rotate your head to the center.

Repeat movement cycles a and b 3 times.

Inhale deeply.

- a. Exhale as you slowly rotate your head to the right while pushing your chin gently with your left hand.

- b. Inhale as you slowly rotate your head to the center.

Repeat movement cycles a and b 3 times.

Relax and breathe into the posture.

Concentrate on your breathing.

Neck Stretch Posture

Sit straight facing forward with your feet together.

Inhale deeply.

Bring your left hand up and around to the right side of your head.

Inhale deeply.

   a. Exhale as you slowly pull your head to the left with your left hand.

   b. Inhale as you slowly bring your head to the center.

Repeat movement cycles a and b 3 times.

Inhale deeply.

   a. Exhale as you slowly pull your head to the right with your right hand.

   b. Inhale as you slowly bring your head to the center.

Repeat movement cycles a and b 3 times.

Relax and breathe into the posture.

Concentrate on your breathing.

Seated Posture With Arms Stretched Up

Sit straight facing forward with your feet together.

Extend your arms along the sides of your body with palms facing your thighs and fingers

pointing down.

    a. Inhale as you raise your arms to the sky with palms facing forward.

    b. Exhale as you allow your shoulders to lower slightly, while keeping your arms vertical.

Repeat movement cycles a and b 3 times.

Relax and breathe into the posture.

Concentrate on your breathing.

Seated Posture With Bound Hands

Sit straight facing forward with your feet together.

Raise your arms just above your head, interlock your fingers and rotate your palms facing up.

    a. Inhale as you push your hands and arms up to the sky.

    b. Exhale as your allow your hands and arms to lower slightly, while keeping your arms vertical.

Repeat movement cycles a and b 3 times.

Relax and breathe into the posture.

Concentrate on your breathing.

Elevated Arm Stretch Posture

Sit straight facing forward with your feet together.

Bring your left arm straight up.

Bend your elbow and allow your left hand to come down behind your head.

Hold your left elbow with your right hand and pull slightly.

    a. Inhale as you slowly lean slightly backward.

    b. Exhale as you slowly lean forward.

Repeat movement cycles a and b 3 times.

Relax and breathe into the posture.

Concentrate on your breathing.

Repeat for the other side.

Posterior Hand Clasp Posture

Sit straight facing forward with your feet together.

Clasp your hands behind your back.

    a. Inhale as you lift your chest.

    b. Exhale as you drop your shoulders and hands.

Repeat movement cycles a and b 3 to 7 times.

Relax and breathe into the posture.

Concentrate on your breathing.

Horizontal Adduction Posture

(Adduction is towards the body, Abduction is away from the body)

Sit straight facing forward with your feet together.

Bring your left arm across your chest parallel to the floor with your palms facing downward.

Bring your right hand to your left arm between your shoulder and elbow.

   a. Inhale as your pull slightly.

   b. Exhale as you slowly release your arm slightly.

Repeat movement cycles a and b 3 times.

Relax and breathe into the posture.

Concentrate on your breathing.

Repeat for the other side.

Seated Cobra Posture

Sit straight facing forward with your feet together.

Place your palms on the seat.

   a. Inhale as you sweep up, arch your back, and tilt your head back if possible.

   b. Exhale as you lower your head down and arch your back down.

Repeat movement cycles a and b 3 times.

Relax and breathe into the posture.

Concentrate on your breathing.

Seated Back Bend Posture

Sit straight facing forward with your feet together and your hand on your hips.

Inhale as you lift your chest and shoulders.

Exhale as you lean back as far as you can go without pain or falling back with your head

gently tilted back.

Inhale deeply.

a. Exhale as you slowly swing your torso in an arc to the left.

b. Inhale as you slowly swing your torso in an arc to the center.

c. Exhale as you slowly swing your torso in an arc to the right.

Repeat movement cycles a, b, and c, 3 times - always returning to center before moving

left or right.

Relax and breathe into the posture.

Concentrate on your breathing.

Seated Leg Elevation Posture

Sit straight facing forward with your feet together.

Place your arms to the side with your palms resting on the seat.

a. Inhale as you slowly raise your legs.

b. Exhale as you slowly lower your legs.

Repeat movement cycles a and b 3 times.

Relax and breathe into the posture.

Concentrate on your breathing.

Seated Spinal Twist Posture

Sit straight facing forward with feet together.

Rotate your torso to the left.

Place your left palm on the seat behind you.

Bring your right hand over your left leg and rest your palm on the seat behind you with your head up.

    a. Inhale as you slowly rotate your torso to the left.

    b. Exhale as you slowly rotate your torso to the center.

Repeat movement cycles a and b 3 times.

Relax and breathe into the posture.

Concentrate on your breathing.

Repeat for the other side.

Seated Forward Fold Posture

Sit straight facing forward with your feet together.

    a. Inhale as you raise your arms straight up to the sky with palms facing forward.

    b. Exhale as you slowly bend forward with your arms down and forward as far as possible while keeping your head down.

Repeat movement cycles a and b 3 times.

Relax and breathe into the posture.

Concentrate on your breathing.

Seated Leg Stretch Posture

Sit straight facing forward with your feet together.

Grasp your right ankle and bend your knee.

    a. Inhale and bring your ankle as far back as possible.

    b. Exhale and release slightly.

Repeat movement cycles a and b 3 times.

Relax and breathe into the posture.

Concentrate on your breathing.

Seated Half Lotus Posture

Sit straight facing forward with your feet together.

Bend your left leg and place your left foot over your right thigh.

    a. Inhale as you raise your knee up.

    b. Exhale as you allow your knee to push down while keeping your head up.

Repeat movement cycles a and b 3 times.

Relax and breathe into the posture.

Concentrate on your breathing.

Repeat for the other side.

Pranic Breathing Meditation

Sit straight facing forward with your feet apart.

Begin meditating by closing your eyes and imagining someone who will help you to feel love. Open your heart and feel love, unconditional love for people, animals, plants, and all of God's creations. Feeling love is the most important part of this meditation.

Imagine that there is a hollow tube about 1-1/2 inches in diameter that extends from the top of your head, through your body along your spine to the bottom of your spine.

Inhale slowly and deeply. Expand your diaphragm and belly first, then allow your chest to expand as you draw in prana through the top and bottom of the hollow tube.

The inhalation should take about 7 seconds.

Exhale slowly and deeply by contracting your diaphragm and belly first, then allowing your chest to contract as you concentrate the prana in your hara (belly).

The exhalation should take about 7 seconds.

Repeat the inhalations and exhalations deeply for 7 breaths. After the 7 deep breathes, begin to breathe normally and regularly.

Concentrate on the regularity of your breathing and the flow of prana through the tube from both directions and the concentration of prana in your hara. It is not unusual to feel palpitation in your heart as the energy flows through your body. This is the life-giving energy that cleanses and rebuilds your mind and body.

As thoughts or pictures come into your mind, allow them to be the focus of your attention. Allow them to enter and exit your consciousness freely.

In meditation, you will meet and melt away emotional and mental blocks, as well as physical tensions. You will generally feel peaceful and refreshed after meditating.

It is beneficial to meditate at least a few times per week. The actual time of each meditation will vary - don't be concerned with time.

In this altered state of consciousness you will be able to be in contact with nature, and the universe around you. The possibilities of what you can do in this state are limitless.

Wheat, Gluten, Dairy, Egg, and Yeast, Free Recipes

Breakfast

Almond Breakfast Cereal or Snack

1/4 cup almond flour

1/4 cup cashew nuts, chopped coarsely

1/4 teaspoon ground cinnamon

Dash of nutmeg

1/8 cup water

Cashew Breakfast Cereal or Snack

1/4 cup almond flour

1/4 cup cashew nuts, chopped coarsely

1/4 teaspoon ground cinnamon

Dash of nutmeg

1/8 cup water

Appetizers

Baba Ghannouj

Preheat oven to 450 degrees F.

2 large eggplants (about 2 pounds)

3 tablespoons cold pressed sesame oil

2 cloves garlic, finely mashed

4 tablespoons sesame seeds

1/2 teaspoon sea salt

1/2 teaspoon black pepper

Peel and grate the eggplants. Bake grated eggplant in a casserole with cover for 45 minutes. Remove from oven and let stand until cool. Simmer garlic in oil a few minutes or until lightly brown. Mix all ingredients with an electric mixer for 1 minute. Place mixture in a bowl, cover and refrigerate for one day. Remove from refrigerator 30 minutes before serving. Serve with vegetables you like except potatoes or carrots

Bean Dip

3 tablespoons cold pressed olive oil

2 cloves garlic, chopped

30 oz. refried beans

3/4 cup water

1/2 teaspoon basil

1/4 teaspoon black pepper

1/2 teaspoon oregano

1/2 teaspoon parsley

1/2 teaspoon sea salt

Using a deep skillet, sauté the garlic in olive oil until dark brown. Lower heat and add remaining ingredients. Cook for another 5 minutes. Serve with vegetables you like except potatoes or carrots

Bean Salad

16 oz. kidney beans, drained

16 oz. garbanzo beans, drained

2 cloves garlic, finely chopped

1/2 cup cold pressed olive oil for dressing

Mix the above ingredients together and serve.

Hummus

16 oz. garbanzo beans
3 tablespoons cold pressed olive oil
1 clove garlic or more, finely mashed
1 teaspoon parsley
dash of cayenne pepper
1/4 cup water

Add garbanzo beans, sesame oil, garlic, cayenne, and 1/4 cup of water to a food processor. Process until smooth. Add more water if mixture is too thick. Allow to chill in the refrigerator for at least one hour. Spread on a flat platter and garnish with parley. Serve with vegetables you like except potatoes or carrots.

Indian Red Relish

2 cloves garlic, chopped
1 onion, chopped (optional)
8 oz. tomato puree
3 tablespoons cold pressed olive oil
1/2 teaspoon cayenne pepper or less
1 teaspoon turmeric
1/2 teaspoon coriander
1/2 teaspoon cumin
1/4 teaspoon salt
1/4 teaspoon black pepper
1/4 cup water

Mix all above ingredients. Serve with vegetables you like except potatoes or carrots.

Salmon Spread

1/2 pound salmon, cooked
3 teaspoons cold pressed olive oil
1/8 teaspoon cayenne pepper
1/2 teaspoon basil
1/4 teaspoon sea salt
1/8 teaspoon black pepper

Blend salmon in food processor. Gradually add oil. Add the remaining ingredients and continue blending until mixture is smooth. Cover and store in refrigerator. Serve chilled.

Soups

Bean and Mushroom Soup

4 tablespoons cold pressed olive oil
2 large cloves garlic, chopped
1/2 tablespoon organic butter
1 bunch scallions, chopped
3/4 pound mushrooms, sliced
4 cups water
1/2 teaspoon sea salt
1/2 teaspoon black pepper
Dash of cayenne pepper
1 tablespoon parsley
1 tablespoon basil
1 tablespoon oregano
2 cans white beans, drained and washed

In a 6-quart pot, sauté the garlic, olive oil, and butter at medium heat until the garlic is lightly brown. Add the scallions and continue to cook for another minute. Add the mushrooms and continue cooking for another 5 minutes. Add the remaining ingredients and simmer for 20 minutes. Remove the pot from the stove and puree the soup with a hand blender. Caution soup is hot. Be very careful while pureeing. Serve hot.

Healthy Chicken Soup

4 cups water

1 pound mushrooms, sliced

1 pound zucchini and yellow squash, cut into medium pieces

12 oz. baby carrots

3 pounds boneless, skinless, chicken tenderloins

10 oz. frozen corn

3 tablespoons oregano

2 tablespoons butter

---

5 oz. baby romaine

1/2 cup cold pressed olive oil

Add all the ingredients above except the romaine and olive oil into an 8 quart pot. Cover and simmer for 1.5 to 2 hours. Stir occasionally. Remove from heat. Add romaine and olive oil. Serve with brown rice or potato

Vegetable Soup

8 cups water (3 quarts)
1 cup brown or green lentils
1 pound mushrooms, sliced
4 stalks celery, sliced
2 cloves garlic, chopped
2 tablespoons parsley
2 teaspoon basil
1/8 teaspoon or more cayenne pepper
1/2 teaspoon black pepper
1 teaspoon sea salt

Bring water to a boil in an 8-quart pot. Add ingredients and allow to a boil for 3 minutes. Lower heat and simmer for 1 hour. Stir occasionally. Serve hot. Leftover soup can be frozen. Serves 6 to 8 people.

Spaghetti Squash Soup

3 tablespoons cold pressed olive oil

2 cloves garlic, chopped

1 spaghetti squash

Chinese cabbage or bok choy (optional)

1 red bell pepper, chopped

1 green bell pepper, chopped

1 onion, chopped (optional)

1/2 pound mushroom, sliced

1 teaspoon sea salt

1/2 teaspoon black pepper

1 teaspoon parsley

1 teaspoon basil

1/2 teaspoon oregano

1/8 teaspoon or more cayenne pepper

Water

Bake the spaghetti squash in an over for 1 hour at 375 degrees F. Remove it from the oven and allow it to cool. Cut the squash in half lengthwise. Remove the seeds. With a fork, strip the strands of squash from the shell.

Sauté garlic in olive oil until lightly brown in an 8-quart pot at medium heat. Add onions, peppers and mushrooms. Continue cooking for about 5 minutes. Add the remaining ingredients. Add water to about 1 inch above the ingredients. Cook for 1 hour at low heat.

Snacks

Zucchini

1 raw zucchini
Cold pressed olive oil
Sea salt
Black pepper
Oregano

Skin the zucchini. Cut it into slices that are about 1/4 inch thick. Lay them out on a plate. Add a few drops of olive oil and other ingredients on top of each. Serve cold.

Mushrooms

Raw button mushrooms
Cold pressed olive oil
Sea salt
Black pepper
Oregano

Cut in half. Lay them out on a plate with the cut side up. Add a few drops of olive oil and other ingredients on top of each. Serve cold.

Vegetables

Any raw vegetables you like except potatoes or carrots
Cold pressed olive oil
Sea salt
Black pepper
Oregano

Cut the vegetables as desired. Lay them out on a plate. Add a few drops of olive oil and other ingredients on top of each. Serve cold.

Sauces

Curry Sauce

3 tablespoons cold pressed olive oil

2 cloves garlic, chopped

16 oz. tomato puree

1/2 teaspoon black pepper

1/2 teaspoon cardamom

A dash or more of cayenne

1 teaspoon turmeric

1/2 teaspoon coriander

1/2 teaspoon cumin

1/4 teaspoon sea salt

Sauté garlic and oil in a 3-quart pot. Add remaining ingredients. Simmer for 10 to 20 minutes.

Marinara Sauce

3 tablespoons cold pressed olive oil
4 large cloves garlic, chopped
1 onion, chopped (optional)
28 oz. whole tomatoes
6 fresh basil leaves, chopped
1 tablespoon oregano
1 tablespoon parsley
1 tablespoon basil
1/2 teaspoon sea salt
1/2 teaspoon black pepper
Dash of cayenne pepper

The origins of marinara sauce, is that the sauce was made in Naples for the sailors when they returned from the sea. The sauce does not contain fish or anything from the sea.

In an 6-quart pot, sauté' garlic and olive oil at medium heat until the garlic is soft and lightly browned. Crush the tomatoes with a fork or puree the tomatoes in a blender. Add remaining ingredients except the basil. Bring to a boil, then lower heat to a simmer and cook until thickened approximately 20 to 30 minutes. Add basil just before serving. Serve over vegetables. Serves 2-4 people.

Garlic and Oil Sauce

3 tablespoons cold pressed olive oil
2 cloves garlic, finely chopped
1 teaspoon parsley
1/2 teaspoon oregano
1/2 teaspoon sea salt
1/8 teaspoon black pepper
1/4 cup soup broth

Sauté garlic until brown; let cool for 2 minutes. Add rest of ingredients and continue cooking for 5-10 minutes. Add vegetables.

Pesto Sauce

2 cups fresh basil leaves
1 cup parsley
1/4 cup cold pressed olive oil
2 cloves garlic, pressed

Mix in a food processor or blender, heat mildly and pour over 1/2 to 1 pound of brown rice or quinoa pasta. Serves 2 people.

Tahini Sauce & Dressing

1 cup sesame tahini
1/2 cup or more water
4 tablespoons cold pressed olive oil
1/2 teaspoon sea salt
1/2 teaspoon black pepper
Mix above ingredients in a blender until smooth. If used as a salad dressing, add more water.

Tomato Sauce

4 tablespoons cold pressed olive oil
2 cloves garlic, chopped
2 onions, chopped (optional)
32 oz. tomato puree
1/2 pound mushrooms, sliced
1 tablespoon oregano
1 tablespoon fresh basil
1 tablespoon parsley
1/2 tablespoon sea salt
1/2 teaspoon black pepper
1/2 teaspoon or less cayenne pepper
6 fresh basil leaves, chopped
1 pound any vegetables you like except potatoes or carrots

In an 8-quart pot sauté garlic in oil until brown. Add remaining ingredients. Simmer 2 hours, stirring every 15 minutes. Serves over vegetables.

Main Dishes

Baked Tilapia

Preheat oven to 350 degrees F.

Fresh tilapia

Cold pressed olive oil

Sea salt

Black pepper

Garlic powder

Oregano

Add a little olive oil to the bottom of a 24-ounce au gratin baking dish or a Pyrex 9.5 x 15.2 x 2.2 inch baking dish. Place the tilapia (3 tilapia in the Pyrex dish) with the side with the red marks, down into the baking dish. Sprinkle some olive oil over the tilapia. Sprinkle some salt, pepper, garlic powder and oregano over the top of the tilapia. Cover with aluminum foil. Bake in the oven at 350 degrees F for 30 minutes. Each tilapia feeds one.

Chicken Creole

3 tablespoons cold pressed olive oil

3 cloves garlic, chopped

2 cloves of garlic, chopped

1 green pepper, chopped

2 pounds chicken breasts, cut into 3/4" pieces

2 stalks of celery, diced

1 large bay leaf

1 teaspoon basil

1/8 teaspoon black pepper

1/8 teaspoon cayenne pepper

1 teaspoon parsley

1/2 teaspoon sea salt

16 oz. tomato puree

2 cups water

Heat oil (high-medium) in deep sauté pan. Sauté garlic for 10 minutes or until brown. Add garlic and green pepper, and continue cooking for another 5 minutes. Add all other ingredients and continue cooking for 10 minutes. Serves 2 to 4 people.

Blackened Tuna

2 tuna filets or steaks

3 tablespoons cold pressed olive oil

2 cloves garlic, chopped

1 teaspoon or more black pepper

1 teaspoon parsley

3 oz. baby romaine

Place the olive oil in a large sauté' pan at medium-high heat. Add the garlic and cook until slightly brown. Push the garlic to the edge around the pan. Add black pepper to both sides of the tuna. Place the tuna in the center of the pan. Add the other spices to everything in the pan. Cook the tuna until it is browned. Turn over and brown the other side. The tuna is done when the center is cooked. Serve over a bed of romaine. Serves two.

Chicken Cacciatore

3 tablespoons cold pressed olive oil

2 cloves garlic, chopped

1 onion, chopped (optional)

32 oz. tomato puree

1 whole chicken cut up in pieces

1 tablespoon oregano

1 tablespoon parsley

1/2 tablespoon sea salt

1/4 teaspoon black pepper

2 basil leaves

1 pound any vegetables you like except potatoes or carrots

Brown garlic in oil in a small fry pan. Put all ingredients together in an 8-quart pot. Simmer 1 hour, stirring every 15 minutes. Serves 4 people.

Chicken Casserole with Crushed Tomatoes

Preheat oven to 350 degrees F.

3 pounds thin sliced chicken breast (about 6 pieces)

2 cloves garlic, finely chopped

28 oz organic crushed plum tomatoes

3 tablespoons cold pressed olive oil

1/4 teaspoon sea salt

1/8 teaspoon fine black pepper

1 teaspoon parsley

6 fresh basil leaves, chopped

1 teaspoon oregano

Dash of cayenne pepper (optional)

Mix the above ingredients, except the chicken, in a bowl. Place a small amount of olive oil on the bottom of a covered Pyrex baking dish. Place the chicken breasts on the bottom of the dish. Pour over some tomato mixture. Add another layer of chicken breasts. Pour over more tomato mixture. Pour the remaining tomato mixture on the top layer. Cover and bake 90 minutes at 350 degrees F. Serves 6 people.

Chili

3 tablespoons cold pressed olive oil

2 cloves garlic, finely chopped

1 onion, chopped (optional)

1 green pepper, chopped

16 oz. tomatoes, finely chopped

16 oz. tomato puree

16 oz. white beans, drained

1 cup water

1 teaspoon basil

1/2 teaspoon black pepper

6 teaspoons chili powder

1 teaspoon oregano

1 teaspoon parsley

1/2 teaspoon sea salt

Heat oil in an 8-quart pot at medium heat. Sauté garlic, and peppers until brown. Add remaining ingredients. Cover and simmer for 60 minutes. Add more water if sauce is too thick. Serves 6 people.

Chopped Meat (Turkey) Allocca Style

2 tablespoons cold pressed olive oil

2 cloves garlic, chopped

1 onion, chopped (optional)

1/2 green pepper, finely chopped

16 oz. tomato puree

1 pound chopped turkey

1 teaspoon oregano

1/2 teaspoon parsley

1/2 teaspoon basil

1/2 teaspoon garlic powder

1/2 teaspoon sea salt

1/8 teaspoon black pepper

Dash cayenne pepper

Sauté garlic. Place remaining ingredients in a 4-quart pot, cover and cook for 10 -15 minutes over a medium heat, stirring frequently. Serve hot. Serves 2 people.

Curry Casserole

3 tablespoons cold pressed olive oil
2 cloves garlic, chopped
1 onion, chopped (optional)
16 oz. tomato puree
16 oz. lentils
1 head broccoli, chopped
1/2 teaspoon sea salt
1/2 teaspoon black pepper
1/2 teaspoon cardamom
A dash of cayenne, to your taste
1 teaspoon turmeric
1/2 teaspoon coriander
1/2 teaspoon cumin

In a 6-quart pot, sauté garlic in oil until slightly brown. Add rice and sauté for another minute. Add remaining ingredients. Bring to a boil. Cover, lower heat, and simmer for 45 minutes.

Healthy Salad

Romaine lettuce
Cabbage, sliced
Red or green pepper, cut up
Bean sprouts
Mushrooms, sliced
Any additional vegetables you like except potatoes or carrots
Cold pressed olive oil for dressing

Kale Casserole

2 tablespoons cold pressed olive oil
2 cloves garlic, chopped
1 onion, chopped (optional)
1 large bunch of kale, chopped
1/2 teaspoon sea salt
1/4 teaspoon black pepper
1 teaspoon basil
1/2 teaspoon parsley
1/2 teaspoon oregano

In a 6-quart pot, sauté garlic in oil until slightly brown. Add rice and sauté for another minute. Add remaining ingredients. Bring to a boil. Cover, lower heat, and simmer for 45 minutes.

Kale with Garlic and Oil

1 pound rice or corn pasta, cooked and drained
2 tablespoons cold pressed olive oil or more
2 cloves garlic, chopped
1 onion, chopped (optional)
1 bunch of kale, cut up
1/2 pound Shitaki mushrooms, sliced
1 teaspoon parsley
1 teaspoon oregano
1 teaspoon basil
1/2 teaspoon sea salt
1/8 teaspoon black pepper

Heat oil in a skillet. Add garlic, and mushrooms. Sauté until mushrooms and garlic are brown. Add remaining ingredients and sauté another 10 minutes. Serve over pasta. Serves 2 to 4 people.

Meat (Turkey) Loaf

Preheat oven to 425 degrees F.

2 tablespoons cold pressed olive oil

2 cloves garlic, chopped

1 onion, chopped (optional)

1 green pepper, chopped

1/2 pound fresh mushrooms, sliced

8 oz. tomato puree

2 pounds lean chopped turkey

1 tablespoon oregano

1/2 teaspoon parsley

1/2 teaspoon black pepper

1/2 teaspoon basil

1/2 teaspoon sea salt

2 teaspoons xantham gum

1/2 teaspoon agar agar

Sauté garlic till brown and put aside. Sauté mushrooms till brown and put aside. Mix all above ingredients except tomato sauce. Make into a load and cover with tomato sauce. Bake in oven at 425 degrees for 60 minutes. Serves 2 to 4 people

Portobella Casserole

2 tablespoons cold pressed olive oil or more
2 cloves garlic, chopped
1 onion, chopped (optional)
1 pound Portabella mushrooms, diced into 3/4" squares
3-1/2 cups water
6 oz. baby romaine
1/2 teaspoon sea salt
1/4 teaspoon black pepper
1 teaspoon basil
1/2 teaspoon parsley
1/2 teaspoon oregano

In a 6-quart pot, sauté garlic in oil until slightly brown. Add mushrooms and sauté for another 5 minutes. Add rice and sauté for another minute. Add remaining ingredients. Bring to a boil. Cover, lower heat, and simmer for 45 minutes.

Roasted Chicken

Preheat oven to 350 degrees F.

Oil the bottom of a large poultry pan with v-shaped rack. Place cut potatoes and carrots on the bottom of the pan. Place cut onions and carrots on top of the potatoes. Sprinkle with cold pressed olive oil, sea salt (small amount), black pepper, parsley, basil, and oregano. Place the chicken on the v-shaped rack. Approximate cooking times are as follows:

3 pounds = 1 hour, 50 minutes

3.5 pounds = 2 hours

4 pounds = 2 hours, 10 minutes

5 pounds = 3 hours

6 pounds = 2 hours, 50 minutes

7 pounds = 3 hours, 10 minutes

8 pounds = 3 hours, 30 minutes

Note: if the chicken(s) were frozen and not fully thawed, add 30 minutes to the cooking time.

The roasting pan recommended is the "Rachael Ray Oven Lovin' Non-Stick 10" x 14" Roaster with V-Rack." The non-stock pan and rack make it is easy to clean. Two 3.5 pound chickens can fit in this pan.

Sausage (Chicken) with Onions and Peppers

2 pounds chicken sausage

2 tablespoons cold pressed olive oil

2 onions, chopped (optional)

2 bell peppers, chopped

1 teaspoon parsley

1 teaspoon oregano

1 teaspoon basil

1/2 teaspoon sea salt

1/8 teaspoon black pepper

In a 6-quart pot, add the oil, onions, and peppers. Cook covered over medium heat for 5 minutes. Add the sausages and continue cooking covered for 20 minutes or until done. Serves 2 to 4 people.

Salmon or Tuna – Allocca Style

2 tablespoons cold pressed olive oil or more
2 cloves garlic, chopped
2 salmon or tuna filets
1/2 teaspoon black pepper
1/4 teaspoon sea salt
1 teaspoon parsley
6 fresh basil leaves, chopped
3 oz. fresh organic baby romaine

Remove the skin from the filet using a paper towel to grip it. Place the olive oil in a large sauté pan at medium-high heat. Add the garlic and cook until slightly brown. Push the garlic to the edge around the pan. Place the salmon filet in the center of the pan. Add basil to the garlic around the edge of the pan. Add the other spices the pan. Cook the salmon until it is browned. Turn over and brown the other side. The salmon is done when the center is white. Serve over a bed of romaine. Serves two.

Stuffed Chicken with Mushrooms

1 pound portabella or button mushrooms, chopped

2 tablespoons cold pressed olive oil

1/2 teaspoon sea salt

1/4 teaspoon black pepper

Dash of cayenne pepper

1/2 teaspoon parsley

1/2 teaspoon basil

1/2 teaspoon oregano

2 cloves garlic, chopped

1 onion, chopped (optional)

3 pounds (10 slices) thin-sliced chicken breast

Sauté mushrooms in oil for 5 minutes. Add herbs and spices and set aside. Place 5 thin-sliced chicken breasts into an oiled 15 x 10 x 2 Pyrex dish. Add some mushroom mixture to each slice. Next, place another 5 thin-sliced chicken breast on top of each of the previously filled breasts. Add the remaining mixture on top of each thin-sliced chicken breast. Place in the oven and low broil for 35 minutes.

Stuffed Chicken with Tomatoes and Olives

16 oz tomato puree

16 oz black olives, chopped

2 tablespoons cold pressed olive oil

1/2 teaspoon sea salt

1/4 teaspoon black pepper

Dash of cayenne pepper

1/2 teaspoon parsley

1/2 teaspoon basil

1/2 teaspoon oregano

1/2 teaspoon garlic powder

3 pounds (10 slices) thin-sliced chicken breast

Mix the tomatoes, olives, herbs, and spices in a bowl and set aside. Place 5 thin-sliced chicken breasts into an oiled 15 x 10 x 2 Pyrex dish. Add some tomato and olive mixture to each slice. Next, place another 5 thin-sliced chicken breast on top of each of the previously filled breasts. Add the remaining mixture on top of each thin-sliced chicken breast. Place in the oven and low broil for 35 minutes.

Turkey

Preheat the oven to 400 degrees F.

Place cut potatoes and place them on the bottom of a large poultry pan with v-shaped rack. Place cut carrots onions on top of the potatoes. Sprinkle with cold pressed olive oil, sea salt (small amount), black pepper, and garlic powder.

Place the turkey on the v-shaped rack.

Make a batter of olive oil, melted butter (small amount), sea salt (small amount), and black pepper. Inject the batter into the turkey.

Make a "tent" out of aluminum foil and place it loosely over the turkey to keep it moist.

Cook the turkey for 1 hour. Lower the temperature to 350 degrees F.

Insert a cooking thermometer into the breast of the turkey. Cook the turkey until it reaches 165 degrees F. Approximate cooking times:

10 pounds = 3 to 3-1/2 hours

15 pounds = 3-1/2 to 4 hours

20 pounds = 4 to 4-1/2 hours (feeds 10 people)

25 pounds = 4-1/2 to 5 hours

30 pounds = 5 to 5-1/2 hours

Remove the aluminum foil tent 1 hour before the turkey is cooked to brown the skin.

Vegetable Casserole

2 tablespoons cold pressed olive oil
2 cloves garlic, chopped
1 onion, chopped (optional)
1 red pepper, chopped
1/2 pound mushrooms, sliced
1 cup lentils, cooked
16 oz. tomatoes, finely chopped
Vegetables, chopped (bok choy, kale, etc.)
1 teaspoon basil
1/2 teaspoon black pepper
Dash of cayenne pepper
1 teaspoon garlic powder
1 teaspoon oregano
1 teaspoon parsley
1 teaspoon sea salt

In a 8-quart pot, sauté garlic, peppers, and mushrooms. Add remaining ingredients. Bring to a boil. Cover and simmer for 45 minutes. Serves 6 to 8 people.

Side Dishes

Baked French Fries

Preheat oven 400 degrees F.

4-5 medium sized potatoes, 2 pounds, washed and dried (do not peel).

Okay, they are not fried. But, they taste great and they are healthy too! Wrap the potatoes in wax paper. Cook in a microwave oven for 1.5 minutes on high. Unwrap and insert each potato into the potato slicer creating french fry cuts. Sprinkle rosemary leaves on top. Place the cuts onto a french fry baking sheet (with holes) and bake in a conventional oven for 45 minutes at 400 degrees F or until golden brown or darker if you prefer.

From www.chefscatalog.com

Progressive Deluxe French Fry Cutter, Item # 26027, $34.95

CHEFS Nonstick French Fry Baking Sheet, Item # 29319, $24.95

Broccoli with Tomato Sauce

2 tablespoons cold pressed olive oil
2 cloves garlic, chopped
1 onion, chopped (optional)
1 large head of broccoli tips
32 oz. tomato puree
1 teaspoon oregano
1 teaspoon parsley
1/2 teaspoon sea salt
1/8 teaspoon black pepper
1 basil leaf

Sauté garlic in oil. Add garlic and brown. Put all ingredients together in a 6-quart pot. Simmer 30 minutes Serve over rice.

Dahl

1 tablespoon cold pressed olive oil
2 cloves garlic, chopped
1/2 cup water or more
1/2 teaspoon black pepper
1/2 teaspoon cardamom
A dash or more of cayenne
1 teaspoon turmeric
1/2 teaspoon coriander
1/2 teaspoon cumin
1/2 teaspoon sea salt
16 oz. lentils

Sauté garlic and oil in a 3-quart pot. Add remaining ingredients. Bring to a boil. Simmer for 30 minutes.

Lentil Salad

Lentils are high in protein and fiber. Fiber will promote bowel movements.

2 cups dry green or brown lentils

4 cups water

1 tablespoon cold pressed olive oil

1/4 teaspoon garlic powder

1/2 teaspoon parsley

1/2 teaspoon basil

1/2 teaspoon oregano

dash of sea salt

dash of black pepper

      Place lentils and water in a 4-quart saucepan. Bring to a boil. Reduce heat, cover, and simmer for 40 minutes or until done. Allow the beans to cool. Then add the remaining ingredients.

Mushrooms in Garlic & Oil

2 tablespoons cold pressed olive oil
2 cloves garlic, chopped
1 onion, chopped (optional)
1 pound shitaki or portabello mushrooms, sliced
1 teaspoon parsley
1 teaspoon oregano
1 teaspoon basil
1/2 teaspoon sea salt
1/8 teaspoon black pepper

Heat oil in a skillet. Add garlic and mushrooms. Sauté until mushrooms and garlic are brown. Add remaining ingredients and sauté another 10 minutes.

Squash

2 pound butternut squash
2 tablespoons cold pressed olive oil
2 cloves of garlic, finely chopped
4 scallions, chopped (optional)
1 leek, sliced
1/2 teaspoon sea salt
1/4 teaspoon black pepper
1 pound rice pasta

Peel the butternut squash. Cut the squash into 4 sections length-wise. Remove the seeds. Slice each section into 1/4" slices. Set aside squash. Begin boiling the water for the pasta. At medium heat, add the garlic to a 6-quart pot and sauté until slightly brown. Add the scallions and cook for another minute. Add the leek and cook for another minute. Add the squash and lower heat. Cover and simmer for 20 to 30 minutes or until the squash is tender. Stir occasionally. Serve separately or over pasta or rice.

Steamed Vegetables

6 pieces of broccoli tips

3 slices of cabbage, cut up

2 pieces of kale, cut up

Any additional vegetables you like except potatoes or carrots

1/2 teaspoon basil

1/2 teaspoon parsley

1/2 teaspoon oregano

1/2 teaspoon sea salt

1 tablespoon cold pressed olive oil

Place potatoes and cabbage in steamer pot and steam for 15 minutes. Add the rest of the ingredients and steam for an additional 5 minutes. For microwave: cover all vegetables and cook for 10 minutes) Add spices as desired.

Stuffed Artichokes

1 tablespoon cold pressed olive oil
2 cloves garlic, finely chopped
6 large-size artichokes
1 teaspoon basil
1 teaspoon parsley
1 teaspoon oregano
1/4 teaspoon sea salt
1/8 teaspoon black pepper

Cut off artichoke stems and trim 1/2 inch from tops of leaves. Separate leaves slightly to allow for stuffing. Sauté garlic and oil until brown. In a large bowl mix together above ingredients. Spoon mixture into the artichokes and place in a steamer pot and steam for 30 minutes at medium heat.

Tossed Salad

Baby romaine
Endive
Radicchio
Garbanzo beans
Cold Pressed Olive Oil for dressing

Use quantities of the above appropriate for the number of people being served.

Bread and Muffins

Banana Nut Muffins

Preheat oven to 350 degrees F.

2 cups brown rice flour

1 cup tapioca flour

2 tablespoons potato starch flour

2 tablespoons baking powder (non-aluminum)

2 tablespoons fructose

2 teaspoons xantham gum

1/2 teaspoon agar agar

1/2 teaspoon sea salt

4 medium fresh almost green bananas, peeled & mashed

3/4 cup almonds or walnuts, chopped

1-3/4 cups rice or coconut milk or water

2 tablespoons cold pressed sunflower oil

1 teaspoon vanilla flavor (non-alcoholic)

Mix dry ingredients with electric mixer. Slowly add the milk while mixing. Add canola oil and vanilla. Add bananas. Spoon mixture into an oiled muffin pan. Bake at 350 F for 45 minutes or until top is light brown. Remove muffins from the pan and cool on a cake rack. Makes 12 muffins.

Blueberry Muffins

Preheat oven to 350 degrees F.

2 cups brown rice flour

1 cup tapioca flour

2 tablespoons potato starch flour

2 tablespoons baking powder (non-aluminum)

3 tablespoons fructose

2 teaspoons xantham gum

1/2 teaspoon agar agar

1/2 teaspoon sea salt

1-3/4 cups rice or coconut milk or water

2 tablespoons cold pressed sunflower oil

1 teaspoon vanilla flavor (non-alcoholic)

1 cup blueberries or other fruit

Mix dry ingredients with electric mixer. Slowly add the milk while mixing. Add canola oil and vanilla. Add blueberries. Spoon mixture into an oiled muffin pan. Bake at 350 F for 40 minutes or until top is light brown. Remove muffins from the pan and cool on a cake rack. Makes 9 muffins. Add a little water to the unused muffin spaces.

Brown Rice Bread

Preheat oven to 350 degrees F.

2 cups brown rice flour

1 cup tapioca flour

2 tablespoons potato starch flour

2 tablespoons baking powder (non-aluminum)

2 tablespoons fructose

2 teaspoons xantham gum

1 teaspoon agar agar

1/2 teaspoon sea salt

1-1/4 cups rice or coconut milk or water

1 tablespoon cold pressed olive oil

Mix dry ingredients with dough hooks. Slowly add the milk while kneading. Add olive oil. Dough will be slightly sticky. Press into an oiled loaf pan with a lightly oiled spatula. Bake at 350 F for 60 minutes or until top is medium brown. Remove from the pan and cool on a cake rack. Variations, add 2 teaspoons of Italian seasoning or other seasoning to your taste.

Brown Rice Foccacia Bread

Preheat oven to 400 degrees F.

1 cup brown rice flour

1/2 cup tapioca flour

1 tablespoon potato starch flour

1 tablespoon baking powder (non-aluminum)

1 tablespoon fructose

2 teaspoons xantham gum

1/2 teaspoon agar agar

1/4 teaspoon sea salt

3/4 cup rice or coconut milk or water

1/2 tablespoon cold pressed olive oil

2 cloves garlic, pressed

    Mix dry ingredients with dough hooks. Slowly add the milk while kneading. Add olive oil. Dough will be slightly sticky. Press into an oiled 8-inch baking pan with a lightly oiled spatula. Brush top with olive oil. Add garlic, salt, pepper, oregano, fresh basil, thinly sliced tomato. Bake at 400 F. for 25 minutes or until crust is medium brown. Remove from the pan and cool on a cake rack.

Corn Muffins

Preheat oven to 350 degrees F.

2 cups yellow corn meal

1/2 cup brown rice flour

1/2 cup tapioca flour

2 tablespoons potato starch flour

2 tablespoons baking powder (non-aluminum)

3 tablespoons fructose

2 teaspoons xantham gum

1/2 teaspoon agar agar

1/2 teaspoon sea salt

1-3/4 cups rice or coconut milk or water

2 tablespoons cold pressed sunflower oil

1 teaspoon vanilla flavor (non-alcoholic)

1 cup corn kernels (optional)

Mix dry ingredients with electric mixer. Slowly add the milk while mixing. Add canola oil and vanilla. Add optional corn kernels. Spoon mixture into an oiled muffin pan. Bake at 350 F for 40 minutes or until top is light brown. Remove muffins from the pan and cool on a cake rack. Makes 9 muffins. Add a little water to the unused muffin spaces.

Desserts

Almond Cookies and Pancakes

Preheat oven to 350 degrees F.

3 cups or cashew almond flour

1 cup cashew nuts - coarsely chopped

1/2 cup sesame seeds

2 teaspoons baking powder (non-aluminum) (2 tablespoons for pancakes)

2 teaspoons ground cinnamon

1 teaspoon ground nutmeg

1/2 teaspoon sea salt

1/2 cup cold pressed sunflower oil

2 teaspoons xantham gum

1/2 teaspoon agar agar

1/4 cup water (1/2 cup for pancakes)

Organic butter to spread

Mix dry ingredients, then add liquids & mix well. Spoon out onto a lightly oiled cookie sheet with a tablespoon or medium size ice cream scoop. Then, flatten slightly. Bake 30 minutes or until slightly brown. Cool on a wire rack. Makes approximately 26 cookies. Turn the cookie upside down and add butter. 7.6 Carbohydrates per cookie (35 g).

Apple Cashew Dessert

3 medium peeled and sliced apples (390 grams, 50.9 grams carbohydrate)

1-1/4 cups filtered water

1 cup cashew nuts (139 grams, 39.7 grams carbohydrate)

1 cup cashew flour (107 grams, 30.6 grams carbohydrate)

4 tablespoons unsweetened shredded coconut (2.3 grams carbohydrate)

4 fresh organic strawberries, sliced

Cinnamon

Place all ingredients into a 4-quart saucepan and cook at medium heat for 10 minutes or until the apples are soft. Place the mixture into four 8 oz pyrex cups. Place one sliced strawberry on top of each cup. Sprinkle cinnamon on top of each cup. Refrigerate and serve cold.

Carbohydrate contents = 130.4 grams divided by 4 = 32.6 grams per serving.

Brown Rice Pudding

1 cup brown rice

1/4 cup fructose

1/4 teaspoon sea salt

2 teaspoons agar agar

1 teaspoon cinnamon

1 teaspoon almond flavor (non-alcoholic)

6 cups rice or coconut milk or water

Place ingredients into a 4-quart pot and bring to a boil. Cover and simmer for 2 hours. Pour into Pyrex cups and refrigerate.

Carrot Cake

Preheat oven to 350 degrees F.

2 cups brown rice flour

1 cup tapioca flour

2 tablespoons potato starch flour

2 teaspoons xantham gum

1 teaspoon agar agar

2 tablespoons baking powder (non-aluminum)

2 teaspoons cinnamon

1 teaspoon salt

1 cup fructose

1/2 cup almonds, chopped

1 cup shredded coconut

2 cups carrots, grated

1 cup cold pressed sunflower oil

1 3/4 cups or more of rice or coconut milk

3 teaspoons almond extract

Combine dry ingredients together. Add liquid ingredients and mix. Add a little water if the mixture is too dry. Put into a 9 x 9 inch oiled pan and bake at 350 F for 45 minutes.

Cashew Cookies and Pancakes

Preheat oven to 350 degrees F.

3 cups cashew flour

1 cup cashew nuts - coarsely chopped

1/2 cup sesame seeds

2 teaspoons baking powder (non-aluminum) (2 tablespoons for pancakes)

2 teaspoons ground cinnamon

1 teaspoon ground nutmeg

1/2 teaspoon sea salt

1/2 cup cold pressed sunflower oil

2 teaspoons xantham gum

1 teaspoon agar agar

1/4 cup water (1/2 cup for pancakes)

Organic butter to spread

Mix dry ingredients, then add liquids & mix well. Spoon out onto a lightly oiled cookie sheet with a tablespoon or medium size ice cream scoop. Then, flatten slightly. Bake 30 minutes or until slightly brown. Cool on a wire rack. Makes approximately 26 cookies. Turn the cookie upside down and add butter. 8.5 Carbohydrates per cookie (35 g).

Coconut Icing

1/2 cup cold pressed sunflower oil

1/2 cup rice or coconut milk

2 tablespoons fructose

1-2 cups shredded coconut (to make thick)

     In a blender, mix all ingredients on high for 3 minutes. Apply to the cake with a spatula.

Pie Crust

Preheat oven to 350 degrees F.

1 cup yellow corn meal

1/4 cup brown rice flour

1/4 cup tapioca flour

1 tablespoon potato starch flour

1 teaspoon baking powder (non-aluminum)

2 tablespoons fructose

2 teaspoons xantham gum

1 teaspoon agar agar

1/4 teaspoon sea salt

1/2 cup rice or coconut milk or water

3 tablespoons cold pressed sunflower oil

1/2 teaspoon vanilla flavor (non-alcoholic)

     Mix dry ingredients with electric mixer. Slowly add rice milk while mixing. Add canola oil and vanilla. Press into an oiled baking pie plate with a lightly oiled spatula. Add filling and bake at 350 F for 50 minutes or until crust is light brown. Allow to cool completely before serving.

Pie Filling - Apple

2 large apples, peeled and sliced

3/4 cup water

1 teaspoon cinnamon

1/2 teaspoon nutmeg

2 teaspoons agar agar

Cover and simmer on low heat for 2 minutes. Add to pie crust.

Pie Filling - Blueberry

16 oz blueberries

3/4 cup water

2 teaspoons agar agar

Cover and simmer on low heat for 2 minutes. Add to pie crust.

Pumpkin Pudding or Pie Filling

2 cups pumpkin or squash, cooked

1/4 cup fructose

1 teaspoon vanilla flavor (non-alcoholic)

1 teaspoon cinnamon

1/2 teaspoon nutmeg

1/2 teaspoon ground ginger

1/4 teaspoon ground cloves

2 teaspoons agar agar

1 cup rice or coconut milk or water

Simmer ingredients in a 4-quart pot. Stir until mixture is well blended. Pour into pyrex cups, then refrigerate. If used as a pie filling, you do not need to simmer the mixture – add to pie crust.

My Own Journey with Migraine

"I suffered from migraine headaches since childhood, spending many nights on the bathroom floor vomiting. In 1995 I tried the so-called miracle drug sumatriptan. I almost had a heart attack from it and it didn't relieve my headache. Furthermore, these drugs have substantial risks. Being a medical scientist, I decided to find a cure for migraine headaches. In 1997 I developed the world's first and only biochemical model of migraine headaches, whereby the exact biochemical mechanisms are revealed. I developed a formula and program to prevent migraine headaches. This is a systemic problem, not only a headache . This formula is safe, effective, and proven in a 2002 study at the Eastern Virginia Medical School. It is a wonderful world without migraine headaches. I can actually make future plans and expect to keep them.

What are you waiting for? Join me on the journey to migraine prevention today! I can work with you in person or by phone, email, and/or postal mail."

Neurotransmitter Solution Analysis and Customized Program

- Analysis and Customized Treatment In-office or by mail

- Consultations by phone and email

Don't Suffer Another Day with Migraine and Other Neurotransmitter Problems

In 1996 Dr. Allocca, a medical scientist and former migraine sufferer, developed a biochemical model revealing the exact mechanisms of action of migraine.

He programmed the migraine and other biochemical models into a computer to analyze a person's biochemical pathways and address complications. The software produces an easy to follow step by step non-drug program, which includes a clinically proven, patented, formula that provides the brain with the nutrients it needs to make neurotransmitters. The formula alone is only part of the program.

Imbalances in brain chemistry, particularly neurotransmitter levels, have a large range of effects on emotions, behavior, brain circulation, and carbohydrate craving.

Neurotransmitters are chemicals that pass signals between the nerves. The neurotransmitters serotonin and norepinephrine send signals through the nerve junctions to the arteries in the brain in order that they may be constricted to a normal diameter against the outward pressure exerted on the walls of the arteries. When there is a loss of neurotransmitters in the brain, there is a loss of signal constricting the arteries, resulting in an enlargement of the arteries, which causes pain and other symptoms.

These neurotransmitter levels in the brain can be diminished by allergic reactions, inflammation, poor absorption of nutrients into the brain, poor metabolism of nutrients in the brain, chemicals that deplete them, excessive depletion (over usage), or insufficient nutrients in the brain to produce enough neurotransmitters. Migraine, depression, insomnia, bipolar disorder, and carbohydrate craving have similar mechanisms and pathways, all resulting from a loss of brain serotonin and norepinephrine.

Migraine, depression, insomnia, bipolar disorder, carbohydrate craving, and more, have similar mechanisms and pathways, all resulting from a loss of the brain neurotransmitters serotonin and norepinephrine.

This customized program for migraine in many cases applies to other areas of brain chemistry imbalance as well.

Tests Analyzed
- Age
- Sex
- Height and Weight
- Blood Pressure
- Temperature
- Urinalysis
- Symptoms Questionnaire

Report / Program
- Vital Statistics
- Basal Metabolic Rate
- Body Mass Index
- Urinalysis Results
- Symptoms Probability Profile
- Conditions which may Interfere with Good Health
- Test Results with Explanations
- Biological Age Factors

- Additional Recommendations
- Food, Supplements, Exercise, and Other Recommendations

You will receive a kit via U.S. Postal Mail. Complete the questionnaire and urine test. Then, return the form to us for processing. We will process your data and return a complete report and plan to you via U.S. Postal Mail. Consultations by phone and email.

Order Your Neurotransmitter Solution Customized Program at www.allocca.com Today!

Brainicity™ Transcranial Neural Network Optimizer

Brainicty™ Transcranial Neural Network Optimizer uses Integrated Harmonic Wave Audio Patterns to:

- Reduce Stress and Anxiety
- Reduce Attention Deficit
- Reduce Headaches
- Reduce Phobias
- Reduce P.T.S.D.
- Help with Epilepsy
- Increase Cognitive Function
- Get Better Sleep
- Increase Performance

Brainicity™ is a safe and drugless system that promotes new neural pathways between the left hemisphere, right hemisphere, and the limbic system of the brain for improved Brain Function, Creativity, and Stress Reduction.

It has long been established that stress is the underlying cause of many diseases. Stress is often not well processed if the brain is lacking neural pathways between the left and right hemispheres. Brainicity™ promotes new neural pathways between the left and right hemispheres of the brain to facilitate the efficient processing of stress and healing.

There is often limited communication between the left and right hemispheres and the limbic system of the brain, which is the emotional center of the brain. If the hemispheres of the brain are utilized separately, they may cope with experiences, especially stressful ones, differently. An internal conflict may be created by different interpretations of the left and right brain hemispheres, potentially resulting in increased anxiety in response to a stressful situation. Without proper communication between the two hemispheres, the conflict may never be resolved and the issue or trauma may become deeply suppressed.

Brainicity™ Binaural uses binaural stimulation whereby different sounds are fed into the left and right ear. The brain perceives a third sound. It is this process that promotes the development of new neural pathways between the right and left hemisphere of the brain.

Brainicity™ Bilateral uses bilateral stimulation whereby sounds are fed into the left and right ears alternately. It is this process that promotes the development of new neural pathways between the right and left hemisphere of the brain.

Just sit back and relax for 21 minutes.

Brainicity™ is available in CD and MP3 formats.

For more information, see
www.allocca.com

References

1. Guyton, A., Textbook of Medical Physiology, tenth edition, W.B. Saunders Company, 2000.

2. Long-term antidepressant treatment decreases spiroperidol-labeled serotonin receptor binding, Peroutka SJ, Snyder, SH, Science, Vol 210, Issue 4465, 88-90, 1980.

3. Orten, J., Neuhaus, O., Human Biochemistry, tenth edition, The C.V. Mosby Co., St. Louis, 1982.

4. Shils, M, Olson, J, Shike, Moshe, Modern Nutrition in health and disease, eighth edition, Lea & Febiger, Pennsylvania, 1994.

5. Mechanism of action of agents used in attention-deficit/ hyperactivity disorder, Wilens, TE, 1: J Clin Psychiatry. 2006;67 Suppl 8:32-8

6. NutriBiotic, 865 Parallel Drive, Lakeport, CA 95453

7. Vitamin Research Products, 4610 Arrowhead Drive, Carson City, Nevada 89706 USA

8. Amino Acid Table, Finnish BodyBuilding Magazine, Bodaus-Issue, February 1997

9. Typical Amino Acid Profile of Whey Protein Powder, Designs for Health, 2 North Road, East Windsor, Connecticut 06088, June 2007.

10. Newer Knowledge of Dairy Foods, Table 16 – Amino Acid Distribution in Milk and Selected Cheeses, National Dairy Counsel, Dairy Management, Inc., Rosemont, Illinois, 60018, 2000.

11. Neuroimaging studies of aggressive and violent behavior: current findings and implications for criminology and criminal justice. Bufkin JL, Luttrell VR., Trauma Violence Abuse. 2005 Apr;6(2):176-91, Drury University, USA.

12. The neural correlates of moral sensitivity: a functional magnetic resonance imaging investigation of basic and moral emotions, Moll J, de Oliveira-Souza R, Eslinger PJ, Bramati IE, Mourão-Miranda J, Andreiuolo PA, Pessoa L., J Neurosci. 2002 Apr 1;22(7):2730-6.

13. Behavioral disinhibition following basal forebrain excitotoxin lesions: alcohol consumption, defensive

aggression, impulsivity and serotonin levels, Johansson AK, Bergvall AH, Hansen S., Department of Psychology, Göteborg University, Sweden, Behav Brain Res. 1999 Jul; 102(1-2):17-29.

14. Low cerebrospinal fluid 5-hydroxyindoleacetic acid concentration differentiates impulsive from nonimpulsive violent behavior, Linnoila M, Virkkunen M, Scheinin M, Nuutila A, Rimon R, Goodwin FK, Life Sci. 1983 Dec 26;33(26):2609-14.

15. The Migraine-Depression Solution, Allocca, John A., Allocca Biotechnology, 2006, ISBN 0-9769213-4-0.

16. The toxic mind: the biology of mental illness and violence, Van Winkle E., Millhauser Laboratories of the Department of Psychiatry, New York University School of Medicine, New York 10016, USA, Med Hypotheses. 2000 Jan;54(1):146-56, Corrected and republished in: Med Hypotheses. 2000 Oct;55(4):356-68.

17. Amino Acid Content of Foods and Biological Data on Proteins, Food Policy and Food Science Service, Nutrition Division, FAO, ISBN 92-5-001102-4, Food and Agriculture Organization of the Untied Nations, Rome – Italy, 1970

18. Crime Times, Vol. 6, No. 4, 2000 Page 1&2

19. Dysfunction in the Neural Circuitry of Emotion Regulation - A Possible Prelude to Violence, Davidson, Richard J, Putnam, Katherine, M, Larson, Christine L, Science 28 July 2000: 591, DOI: 10.1126/science.289.5479.591

20. Raine, the author of The Psychopathology of Crime: Criminal Behavior as a Clinical Disorder, Raine, Adrian, Academic Press, 1993.

21. Dopamine and serotonin: influences on male sexual behavior, Hull EM, Muschamp JW, Sato S., Department of Psychology, University at Buffalo, State University of New York, Buffalo, NY 14260-4110, USA. hull@psy.fsu.edu

22. Impact of single neonatal serotonin treatment (hormonal imprinting) on the brain serotonin content and sexual behavior of adult rats., Csaba G, Knippel B, Karabélyos C, Inczefi-Gonda A, Hantos M, Tekes K, Molecular Immunobiological Research Group, Department of Genetics, Cell and Immunobiology, Semmelweis University of Medicine, POB 370, Budapest H-1445, Hungary. csagyor@dgci.sote.hu

23. Depressed patients have higher body temperature: 5-HT transporter long promoter region effects, Rausch JL, Johnson ME, Corley KM, Hobby HM, Shendarkar N, Fei Y, Ganapathy V, Leibach FH, Neuropsychobiology. 2003;47(3): 120-7, Department of Psychiatry and Health Behavior,

Veterans Administration, The Medical College of Georgia, Augusta, GA 30912, USA. jeffreyr@mail.mcg.edu

24. Human taste thresholds are modulated by serotonin and noradrenaline, Heath TP, Melichar JK, Nutt DJ, Donaldson LF,J Neurosci. 2006 Dec 6;26(49):12664-71, Department of Physiology, University of Bristol, Bristol BS8 1TD, United Kingdom.

25. Role of cholecystokinin and central serotonergic receptors in functional dyspepsia, Chua AS, Keeling PW, Dinan TG, World J Gastroenterol, 2006 Mar 7;12(9): 1329-35.

26. Regional differences in expression of TPH-1, SERT, 5-HT(3) and 5-HT(4) receptors in the human stomach and duodenum, van Lelyveld N, Ter Linde J, Schipper ME, Samsom M., Neurogastroenterol Motil. 2007 May;19(5): 342-8, Gastrointestinal Research Unit, Department of Gastroenterology, University Medical Centre Utrecht, Utrecht, The Netherlands. n.vanlelyveld@azu.nl

27: Acute tryptophan depletion alters gastrointestinal and anxiety symptoms in irritable bowel syndrome, Shufflebotham J, Hood S, Hendry J, Hince DA, Morris K, Nutt D, Probert C, Potokar J, Am J Gastroenterol. 2006 Nov; 101(11):2582-7. Epub 2006 Oct 4. Clinical Science at South Bristol, University of Bristol, Bristol, United Kingdom.

28. The 25th Anniversary of the Prosper Meniere Society – The 12th International Symposium and Workshop on Inner Ear Medicine and Surgery, March 11-14, 2006, Zillertal, Austria.

29. The effects of melatonin on tinnitus and sleep, Megwalu UC, Finnell JE, Piccirillo JF, Otolaryngol Head Neck Surg. 2006 Feb;134(2):210-3. Clinical Outcomes Research Office, Department of Otolaryngology-Head and Neck Surgery, Washington University School of Medicine, St. Louis, Missouri, USA.

30. Fibromyalgia and the serotonin pathway, Juhl JH, Altern Med Rev, 1998 Oct;3(5):367-75

31. Fibromyalgia syndrome and serotonin, Alnigenis MN, Barland P, Clin Exp Rheumatol. 2001 Mar-Apr;19(2):205-10, Division of Rheumatology, Department of Medicine, Albert Einstein College of Medicine, Bronx, New York, USA. Muyessera@hotmail.com

32. 5-Hydroxytryptophan: a clinically-effective serotonin precursor, Birdsall TC, Altern Med Rev. 1998 Aug;3(4): 271-80, 73541.2166@compuserve.com

33. A placebo-controlled study of the effects of L-tryptophan in patients with premenstrual dysphoria, Steinberg S, Annable L, Young SN, Liyanage N, Adv Exp Med Biol.

1999;467:85-8, Department of Psychiatry, McGill University, Montréal, Québec, Canada.

34. Acute tryptophan depletion aggravates premenstrual syndrome, Menkes DB, Coates DC, Fawcett JP, J Affect Disord. 1994 Sep;32(1):37-44, Department of Psychological Medicine, University of Otago, Dunedin, New Zealand.

35. Epidemiology, etiology, and natural treatment of seasonal affective disorder, Miller AL, Altern Med Rev. 2005 Mar;10(1): 5-13, Thorne Research, Inc., PO Box 25, Dover, ID 83825, USA. alanm@thorne.com.

36. Tryptophan depletion: a predictor of future depressive episodes in seasonal affective disorder?, Neumeister A, Habeler A, Praschak-Rieder N, Willeit M, Kasper S, Int Clin Psychopharmacol. 1999 Sep;14(5):313-5, Department of General Psychiatry, Vienna University, Austria. alexander.neumeister@akh-wien.ac.at

37. L-tryptophan augmentation of light therapy in patients with seasonal affective disorder, Lam RW, Levitan RD, Tam EM, Yatham LN, Lamoureux S, Zis AP, Can J Psychiatry. 1997 Apr;42(3):303-6, Department of Psychiatry, University of British Columbia, Vancouver. rlam@unixg.ubc.ca

38. 5-Hydroxytryptamine release from platelets by different red wines: implications for migraine, Pattichis K, Louca LL, Jarman J, Sandler M, Glover V, Eur J Pharmacol. 1995 Jan

13;292(2):173-7, Department of Chemical Pathology, Queen Charlotte's Hospital, London, UK.

39. Effects of Antihistamines on 3,4-Methylenedioxymethamphetamine-Induced Depletion of Serotonin in Rats, S.Y. YEH,1 C. DERSCH,2 R. ROTHMAN, 2 AND J.L. CADET1, SYNAPSE 33:207–217 (1999) , Molecular Neuropsychiatry Section, National Institute on Drug Abuse, Intramural Research Program, National Institute of Health, Baltimore

40. Neurochemical profile of effects of 28 neurotoxic chemicals on the central nervous system in rats (1). Effects of oral administration on brain contents of biogenic amines and metabolites., Kanada M, Miyagawa M, Sato M, Hasegawa H, Honma T, Ind Health. 1994;32(3):145-64, Department of Occupational Diseases, National Institute of Industrial Health, Kawasaki, Japan.

41. Psycho- and Vasoactive Compounds in Food Substances, Walter Lovenberg, Symposium on Toxic Proteins and Peptides, J. Agr. Food Chem., Vol. 22, No. 1, 1974.

42. Serotonin and alcohol intake, abuse, and dependence: findings of animal studies, LeMarquand D, Pihl RO, Benkelfat C, Biol Psychiatry. 1994 Sep 15;36(6):395-421,

Department of Psychology, McGill University, Montréal, Québec, Canada.

43. Brain Serotonin Metabolism during Water Deprivation and Hydration in Rats, N.K. Popova, L.N. Ivanova, T.G. Amstislavskaya, N.N. Melidi, K.S. Naumenko, L.N. Maslova and V.V. Bulygina, Neuroscience and Behavioral Physiology Volume 31, Number 3 / May, 2001, Siberian Division, Russian Academy of Sciences, Institute of Cytology and Genetics, 10 Lavrent'ev Prospekt, 630090 Novosibirsk, Russia

44. Increase in prefrontal cortex serotonin 2A receptors following estrogen treatment in postmenopausal women, Kugaya A, Epperson CN, Zoghbi S, van Dyck CH, Hou Y, Fujita M, Staley JK, Garg PK, Seibyl JP, Innis RB, American Journal of Psychiatry 2003; 160: 1522-4, Department of Psychiatry, Yale University, New Haven, Conn 06516, USA.

45. Influences of serotonin and testosterone in aggression and dominance: convergence with social psychology," Paul C. Bernhardt, Current Directions in Psychological Science, Vol. 6, No. 2, April 1997, pp. 44-48. Address: Paul C. Bernhardt, Department of Educational Psychology, MBH 327, University of Utah, Salt Lake City, UT 84112.

46. Influence of progesterone on serotonin metabolism: a possible causal factor for mood changes, Ladisich W, Psychoneuroendocrinology. 1977;2(3):257-66

47. Ammonia production by intestinal bacteria: the effects of lactose, lactulose and glucose, Vince AJ, Burridge SM, J Med Microbiol. 1980 May;13(2):177-91.

48. Ammonia, the GABA Neurotransmitter System, and Hepatic Encephalopathy, Jones E.A, Metabolic Brain Disease, Volume 17, Number 4, December 2002 , pp. 275-281(7)

49. Molybdenum for Candida Albicans Patients and Other Problems, Dr. George Miroff, Dr. Richard Mowles, Jon B.Pangborn,, William H. Philpott, M.D./Responsible editor/ writer Walter H., Schmitt, Jr., D.C., The Digest of Chiropractic Economics, 31:4, January-February, 1991, pp. 56-63, 29229 Six Mile Road, Livonia, Michigan 48152-3661.

50. Effects of Neurobiology Formula on the Headaches of Chronic Migraineurs" Erin E. Icenbice, PA-S-Investigator, and Patricia Shull, PA-C, Co-Investigator Eastern Virginia Medical School, Norfolk, VA, June 2002.